CONTENTS

Foreword   v

Acknowledgements   vii

Introduction   xi

1   Myths and hard facts about writing for publication   1

2   Identifying your topic   11

3   Knowing your journals   23

4   Approaching an editor   35

5   Planning your article   47

6   Writing your article   57

7   More things to do before publication   77

8   Things to do after publication   89

9   How to be a regular   97

10   How to be funny   113

11   How to turn your dissertation into an article   123

12   How to get a book contract   135

13   How to write that book   155

14   Top tips for success   165

Appendix A   Assessment of some current journals   173

Appendix B   Reminders about punctuation   175

Appendix C   Referencing   177

Appendix D   Suggested templates for articles   181

Appendix E   Proof correction symbols   185

Appendix F   A quick guide to the Internet and the World Wide Web   193

Appendix G   Sample record sheet for writing income   195

Index   197

FOREWORD

How can a profession demonstrate its contribution, or an organisation its competence, or an individual her commitment, innovation and imagination? The answer to all of these is 'with difficulty', in the absence of a body of literature by which our peers and the public can come to know about our work.

We are now at a time of great opportunity, growth in professional journals, and a greatly enhanced academic underpinning to the professions. What remains problematic can be the ability of practitioners, in clinical, academic, educational or management practice, to write clearly, succinctly and illuminatingly for publication.

There is no requirement that says we must write. But increasingly I perceive amongst the practitioners I meet a hunger for knowledge, matched by a desire to record their own personal or team activity, in order to share knowledge and experience, and learn from this. The desire to write must then be put into action in a form that is publishable. This book seeks to assist the aspirant author by providing clear guidance, and demystifying the process. It also provides important advice on what not to do: for example, an unabridged copy of a worthy but lengthy dissertation is unlikely to find favour with most editors!

Professional practice is an iterative process, in which reading about the research and development or practice approaches of others, and sharing our own experience, is crucial.

I hope that many excellent articles, and indeed books, will emerge as a consequence of reading this helpful and timely publication.

Alison Norman CBE HonDSci RGN RM RHV
October 1999

Acknowledgements

I would like to thank Daniel Allen, Clare Parker and Judith Podmore for providing the editors' 'words of wisdom' for this book. I am also very grateful to John Naish, who published my first articles and encouraged me to write more, so setting me on the path to writing this book.

To my daughters, Kayt and Jessi, whose childhood was punctuated by my articles, and who are the sweetest of my successes.

INTRODUCTION

If you are reading this book, you have probably already thought about why you might want to write for publication. However, in case you are still wavering, there are plenty of good reasons why you should write. It is advantageous for your professional development, it looks good on your CV, it might help you to get a job you want, and it might help other nurses in their jobs – so ultimately it might even be good for patients.

Then there are the real reasons why many nurses write – the three Fs. They write for the fun, the fame and the fee. It is a good feeling to produce a well-crafted article – as good as passing a nasogastric tube first time, or getting a hug from a previously intractable client. There is a great buzz to having your name recognised, and hearing people say 'I saw your article last week'. And, of course, while no one ever cruised the Mediterranean on the money they made from writing articles, it is nice to have the extra income to treat yourself now and again.

This book is aimed at nurses and other health professionals who want to write about their professional practice. No matter what stage you are at in your career, from student to retired expert, you have something to contribute to the store of professional knowledge, experience or anecdote.

This book will be helpful if you have written a few pieces before, but want to make writing a regular activity, or if you have never written before, but want or need to start. It focuses first on writing articles for professional journals (the easiest and most lucrative form of writing for the busy professional). It covers all forms of writing, ranging from clinical and educational articles to humorous pieces, regular columns and oddments such as quizzes. The later chapters look at writing a book, including how to plan it, how to prepare the proposal for the publishers and how to set about the actual writing.

The 'workbook' approach is designed to make writing your article a more straightforward task. Each chapter takes you through one step of a logical, foolproof process for producing a publishable article. By the time you have finished reading this book, if you have also completed the 'Write as you read' tasks, you will probably already have a letter of acceptance from a journal for your article.

Is it really that easy? Not exactly. Writing does require considerable time, effort and commitment, without which even highly articulate and literate people fail to get published. Hoewver, if you are willing to invest the time and effort, you can get an article published even if writing does not come easily to you.

The reason this book makes getting published easier is that it is based on my own mistakes. Over the last 10 years I must have made every mistake possible, irritated editors all over the country, and raised the blood pressure of nurses up and down the land. What I have learned from doing this is distilled into this book, to save you time, trouble and embarrassment.

Enjoy the reading, and enjoy the writing.

Rosemary Cook
October 1999

CHAPTER ONE

MYTHS AND HARD FACTS ABOUT WRITING FOR PUBLICATION

Many people think they ought to write something for publication in their professional journals. Indeed, many of them intend to write something – one day. Fewer will actually try to write, and a few of those will get to the end of the process and produce a publishable article. Between those who think they ought to write, and those who actually do so, lies a set of myths about the business of writing which stops many potential authors in their tracks. It is essential that we dispose of some of these myths before setting out to write an article.

THE MYTHS

Some of the commonest myths, frequently cited as a reason for not starting to write, or for giving up early in the process, are as follows:

- 'you have to write about something new, "leading edge" or different'
- 'the journals are swamped with material for publication – I don't stand a chance'
- 'it's not worth writing for the weekly comics'
- 'you can write an article and then send it on the rounds of the journals'
- 'if an article is rejected by one journal, it is a waste of time sending it to another'
- 'the most important thing is how well you write'
- 'I don't have time to go through the process of getting something published'.

THE REALITY

Myth 1: 'you have to write about something new, "leading edge" or different'

A look through any current edition of a professional journal will show you that this is not the case. Certainly some articles are about new developments in practice, or new treatments, but the majority are not. Rather, they are about disease conditions, or professional issues, or patient experiences, which are basically unchanging. Take the issue of *Nursing Standard* which was published as I wrote this chapter. The main contents are shown in Box 1.1. There are topical issues in the news and some in the features, but the majority of the clinical articles are on ageless topics which recur over the years because they are always of interest to nurses.

Box 1.1: Content of current issue of *Nursing Standard*

Professional topics	**Clinical topics**	**Other topics**
Stress in nursing	Nutrition in primary care	Writing a CV
Racism in nursing	Teenagers in hospital	Other careers
Safety in the workplace	Fractured neck of femur	Network
Performance-related pay	Independent care homes	contacts
Essence of nursing		Student nurses
PREP* queries		

*Post-registration Education and Practice

Of course, there is often a particular reason why such articles appear in the journals at a particular time. They may be part of an educational revision series, or their topic may be a focus of concern because of recent adverse publicity. In the next chapter we shall examine more closely how and why articles on the perennial topics get published. For now, remember that:

☞ **A topic does not have to be new to be published.**

Myth 2: 'the journals are swamped with material for publication'

Any journal editor will tell you that they may sometimes receive a lot of paper, but they are seldom swamped with articles suitable for publication! As someone who referees articles submitted to a range of professional journals, I can vouch for the fact that a great deal of material is not presented in a way that can even be considered for publication. Add to that a frustratingly high percentage of authors who are asked to revise their material but do not do so, and it becomes apparent that editors are sometimes very short of suitable material to publish. The weekly journals have a large amount of space to fill over 52 weeks every year, and they are always keen to receive articles from new authors. Note that most of the journals publish 'Guidelines for contributors' in almost every edition for a reason! The more specialist journals have a smaller readership, and an even smaller pool of people who write on the specialist topic, so they are often particularly keen to encourage people to submit articles. In short, remember that:

☞ **Editors want material to publish as much as you want to be published!**

Myth 3: 'it's not worth writing for the weekly comics'

This is a common misconception, and an insulting one at that! Editors, journalists and freelance writers work extremely hard to produce topical, educational and interesting weekly journals, under the pressure of very tight deadlines. You may call them 'magazines' rather than journals, but avoid even thinking of them as 'comics'!

If you are looking for academic credibility through publication, the weekly publications may not be the place for your article. Most of them do now have a system of peer review for clinical articles, but other journals are more highly regarded in academic circles. Matching your material to the right journal is discussed further in Chapter 3.

There are several very good reasons for targeting the weeklies with your first articles:

- the weekly journals have a lot of space to fill, so you may have a greater chance of acceptance, provided that the quality of your material is high
- the weeklies have the highest rate of circulation, so your published article will reach more people
- the weekly journals cover the whole range of clinical and professional topics, so whatever area you work in or want to write about, they will probably want to publish articles on that subject. In addition to the main journal, *Nursing Times* and *Nursing Standard* both have 'sister' publications targeting specific areas of practice, such as community nursing, so you can address a specialist audience even through a generalist magazine (*see* Appendix A for a more detailed analysis of some major UK nursing and health care journals)
- because of their size, the weekly journals have a number of section editors, who are usually only too willing to give specific guidance to an author to ensure that they get the material they need to fill their section
- they include humorous and 'opinion' pieces, as well as clinical and professional articles, so you can try out different styles of writing
- most nurses read them! It may be fashionable to regard the weeklies as less profes-

sionally 'valuable' than the more academic publications, but the weeklies are the journals people have on subscription or circulate on the ward.

Most nurses who write had their first articles published in one or other of the weekly nursing magazines. The latter provide excellent opportunities for all kinds of writing, on all kinds of topics. In short:

☞ **The weekly nursing journals are a great place to start publishing articles.**

Myth 4: 'you can write an article and then send it on the rounds of the journals'

No, you can't! *Never* send an article on the rounds. There are so many reasons not to do this that it is difficult to know where to start. A few examples are listed below.

- An article will only be published if it 'fits' the journal in terms of size, subject matter, approach, timing, level, and so on. The probability of the same article fitting into more than one journal without at least some revision is very small.
- If an article is rejected by the first journal, for which it was originally written, it is bound to be even less suitable for a journal which was not first choice for it, so its chances of rejection steadily increase, while your self-esteem falls lower with each rejection letter.
- Journal editors will quickly recognise a second-hand (or third- or fourth-hand) submission from the style and content, even if you print a fresh copy from your computer each time. In addition to inviting rejection, this will seriously damage your reputation with these editors.
- If the first journal asked for some revisions, these are unlikely to be overlooked by the second journal editor. Sending an article to a different journal is not a way to avoid putting in the work that is needed to make your article publishable.
- There are people (like me) who review articles for a number of different journals, and who will recognise return customers (*see* Box 1.2)!

This might sound very obvious, but it is still depressingly common to hear people say that they are going to write up their project, idea or study and 'send it on the rounds'. Why waste time and annoy good editors when you can greatly increase your chances of publication by a little judicious targeting and adapting? Chapters 2 and 3 will look more closely at targeting your material to a particular journal. Meanwhile, remember:

☞ *Never* send an article 'on the rounds'.

Myth 5: 'if an article is rejected by one journal, it is a waste of time sending it to another'

The experience described in Box 1.2 might seem to support this argument. However,

> **Box 1.2: The manuscript merry-go-round**
>
> I once reviewed an article three times, for three different journals. It was an interesting and well-written account of a topical project, which only required a little additional information and some simple style changes for me to recommend publication. Instead, it turned up, unchanged, on three different editors' desks, for increasingly unsuitable publications. Each time I reviewed it I made the same comments. It was eventually published with some changes, but it could have been out months earlier if the author had been willing to put in the relatively small amount of work required to revise it at an earlier stage of the process.

that author wasted time by sending the same article to different journals. In this example, when revisions have been suggested by a reviewer, the trick is not to send the rejected article *unaltered* to another journal.

In some cases the reason for rejection is not that the article needs revision. In fact, if revision is requested, this is not 'rejection' at all, but 'conditional acceptance'. If the revisions are carried out to the satisfaction of the reviewer and/or editor, the article will be published (for more on this, *see* Chapter 7). However, an article can be rejected by a journal for many other reasons that are unrelated to the style of writing, the suitability of the subject matter for the journal, or the quality of the writing. For example:

- the journal may recently have published an article on the same topic (*see* Chapter 3)
- they may already have an article on the same subject in the pipeline (*see* Chapter 4)
- they may want to use in-house journalists to cover the topic, rather than take an article from a freelancer.

In all of these instances, rejection of your article does not mean that it is badly written, irrelevant or uninteresting. It would definitely be worth making the necessary alterations to target your article at another journal, rather than giving up. Remember:

☞ **Rejection is part of the process, not the end of the process!**

Myth 6: 'the most important thing is how well you write'

This is certainly not the case. If an article is promising because it is the right subject for the right journal, or it describes something which will be of interest to readers, then editors and their staff will go to a great deal of trouble to make it publishable. Editors edit, and sub-editors adapt to house style, cut to fit the space available and correct grammatical errors – you may think that your written English is impeccable,

but even so it is unlikely to reach the published page without some in-house alterations. Of course, you need to submit an article which is as grammatically and techni-
cally correct as you can make it, in order to make the best possible impression on the
editor receiving it, and to minimise the work that needs to be done by the journal
staff. Computer word-processing software can sometimes help with both spelling and
grammar (*see* Box 1.3). Punctuation is a common bugbear, and some useful reminders are listed in Appendix B. However, if these aspects of writing are not your strong
points, do the best you can and then submit the article anyway. If the content is
strong, the rest can be made to follow. The key point to remember is:

☛ **Don't let concern about your writing ability prevent you from submitting interesting and relevant articles to the journals.**

Box 1.3:   Spelling and grammar correction on software programs

Word-processing software always contains a 'spell-checker' facility. Use it, but
don't rely on it completely. It will draw your attention to actual mistakes, but
will not detect when you have used an alternative form of a word in the wrong
context (e.g. 'their' and 'there'). Also, having told you that you have made a
mistake, it then relies on you to choose the correct alternative from the list it
offers. When you have finished the computerised spelling check, read through a
hard copy, on which inappropriate words or forms will be more obvious.
Another important issue to be aware of with computerised spell-checking is that
of American English versus British English. Some journals or publishers ask for
American English spellings (e.g. 'specialize' rather than 'specialise', 'center'
rather than 'centre'). Your computer spell-checker can be set to work with
either, but make sure that you are in the right dictionary! Software grammar
checks can be quite sophisticated. For example, the latest version of Word will
underline questionable grammar in the text, and offer helpful (if sometimes
pedantic) suggestions for improvement. It is usually sensible to act on them.
Don't worry too much about the finer points of grammar, though, as editors and
sub-editors will also be cutting and correcting, and may well (in your opinion)
make things more eccentric rather than less so.

Myth 7: 'I don't have time to go through the process of getting something published'

If I had a pound for every time I have heard this said, I would stop buying lottery
tickets and retire immediately! Very few of the nurses who write regularly for the
nursing journals do so as a full-time occupation. The vast majority are working full-
time in the profession, or combining part-time work with work in the home. Time is
almost infinitely elastic. If you want to be published, you will be able to make the

time to write the article. Bear in mind the following points.

- Opinion pieces are not to be despised, as they often contribute significantly to debates on clinical and professional issues. They are often only 200–500 words long, so can be written relatively quickly.
- Longer articles are always broken up into sections by subtitles. Each section can be written separately using brief bursts of writing time.
- Essential tasks, such as identifying precise subject matter, planning the article, deciding on the subheadings and writing the summary, can be undertaken away from the computer or desk, e.g. on train journeys, in front of the cooker, or while breastfeeding!
- In some cases much of the substance of the article will already have been written in another form, such as a project report or academic assignment (*see* Chapter 11).

Remember:

☛ **Never use time as an excuse for not being published. Time is elastic.**

THE HARD FACTS

Having disposed of some of the many myths surrounding writing for publication, it is time to face some of the hard facts.

Your material has to fit the journal, not the other way round

This applies both to actual fit, in terms of word length, and to content. If the Guidelines for Contributors say that a journal wants articles between 1500 and 2000 words in length, it is pointless to send in a 3500 word article because you feel you cannot do justice to your subject in less space. The journal will either reject it or ask you to cut it. They have to fit in other features, advertisements and regular sections, and they will not redesign the whole journal to accommodate your article. Similarly, the content has to be appropriate. For example, a journal that does not normally publish humorous material will not make an exception for your piece, however good it may be. Send it to a publication that uses such material, otherwise you will be wasting your time and damaging your reputation.

☛ **Choose the right publication and keep to the given word length!**

Other people will write about your topic if you don't

Of course they will not be writing about your specific project or study. However, there will be many other people around the country working in the same clinical area, and sooner or later some of them will write about the topic from the same perspective as your work. If you want to write about your experience of introducing a new treatment for wounds, or setting up multidisciplinary clinical supervision, start your article as soon as possible. There will be a time lag between acceptance and publication in any case, and the longer you wait the more likely it is that your article will be rejected because a journal has already published several other articles on the topic. You will then need to find a new slant, or a reason for making your article particularly topical, in order to find a publisher (*see* Chapter 2).

☞ **If you want to write about something, do it now!**

You cannot make multiple submissions

This can be divided into two hard facts. First, you must not send the same manuscript to more than one journal at once. It might seem like a good idea to save time, given that it can take 3 months to receive a rejection letter, but it is considered unethical. In practical terms, if the article is good enough for publication, and targeted at two similar journals, it may be accepted by both, and then you will be in the unhappy position of having to withdraw it from one of them. Once found out, you are unlikely to have another article considered. The second hard fact is that you cannot offer an article which has been published in one journal to any other journal. You will have signed over copyright of your article to the first journal, precisely (from the journal's point of view) to ensure that they have exclusive rights to publish it. Editors of other journals would not normally want to publish material that has already appeared somewhere else, and generally make it a condition of submission that the material has not been published elsewhere. This does not mean that you cannot write another article based on the same material (*see* Chapters 2 and 11).

☞ **Send your article to one journal at a time, and once it is published, stop!**

Articles will be rejected for many reasons other than lack of merit

This relates directly to the myth that a rejected article is fit only for the waste-paper bin. An article can be rejected because the timing is wrong, because the journal has already published a number of articles on the topic, because they have already commissioned someone else to write on the subject, or because they feel that the subject is not tailored to their readership. This does not mean that it is not a good article. However, rejection is a fact of life for all writers of articles, and should be regarded as a normal part of the process of getting published.

☞ **Do not let rejection stop you writing or submitting articles.**

Journals exist to make money for or raise the profile of their publishers, to attract readers and outdo their rivals

Journals are not in business to develop the nursing profession, protect patients or develop new writers. They frequently do all of these things along the way, but you cannot count on this. The articles they choose to publish, the way in which they cut and edit them, and the prominence that they give them will all be decided in the best interests of the journal, not of the author or the profession. For example, do not expect the journal to protect you from controversy over your opinions or your approach as presented in your article. They may have chosen to publish it precisely in order to generate correspondence to the letters page, and further contributions to the opinion columns. As your name is on the article, you will have to deal with the consequences (*see* Chapter 8).

☛ **Remember that the journals are principally in business to promote themselves, not to protect their authors.**

SUMMARY

Many nurses, midwives and health visitors who could write for the professional journals are reluctant to start, or discouraged from continuing to write, because they subscribe to some of the many myths that surround writing for publication. Once you have made up your mind to disregard these myths, and accepted the hard fact that if you don't get on with writing, someone else will, then you are ready to start writing your next article.

WRITE AS YOU READ 1.1

Check the list of myths at the beginning of this chapter. Which of them have you subscribed to in the past? If you are going to complete this workbook, and produce your publishable article, you need to accept that your particular bugbear myth is untrue. If it helps, write down a positive statement to remind you of this and put it above your desk or on your computer. For example:

- I can make time to write this article
- I am writing for the weekly journal which 90% of the profession read
- It doesn't matter if it isn't perfectly written, because I'm describing a really important project
- I will target and revise my article until it is published.

Similarly, which of the hard facts about writing do you find most difficult to accept?

Again, you need to acknowledge the way things are, even if you don't think this is right, if you are going to find the motivation to complete a publishable manuscript. Be clear in your own mind that you are going to deal with the real world, with all its imperfections, in order to achieve what you want, namely a published article.

CHAPTER TWO

IDENTIFYING YOUR TOPIC

It makes my day if someone comes up with a really innovative idea for an article. Something written from their experience, on a really nitty-gritty area, not just a textbook approach. Something that gets to grips with the issue.

(Clare Parker, Features Editor, 'Practice Nurse')

If you are reading this book with a view to writing something for a professional journal, you may already have a particular topic in mind for your article. In this case, you are already at step 2 on the 'writing ladder' shown in Figure 2.1. This chapter will help you with the essential step of defining and refining that idea before you go any further. Of course it is tempting, when you know what you want to write about, to sit down and write without further ado. You may be impatient to start an article on 'our new day-case unit', 'problem patients in GP surgeries' or 'aromatherapy in labour'. However, trying to leap straight to steps 6 or 7 – planning or writing the article – may save some time at this stage, but will greatly decrease your chance of being published. You are very likely to find yourself returning to steps 3, 4 and 5 eventually, in order to try to remedy the situation at a later stage. This is annoying, demoralising and downright boring! There are some very good reasons for spending time at this stage on refining your idea.

- It is difficult to construct a writing plan for the article unless you are very clear what kind of article it is, how much technical, research, personal or other information you want to include, and the target readership.
- It is impossible to target a suitable journal for your article unless you are absolutely clear what kind of article it is, and who the target readership is – and if you don't target, you are much less likely to get published!

- You will need to be able to 'sell' your idea to the editor (*see* Chapter 4), who will question you about it. If you don't sound clear and confident about what you are going to write and why, you are unlikely to convince him or her.

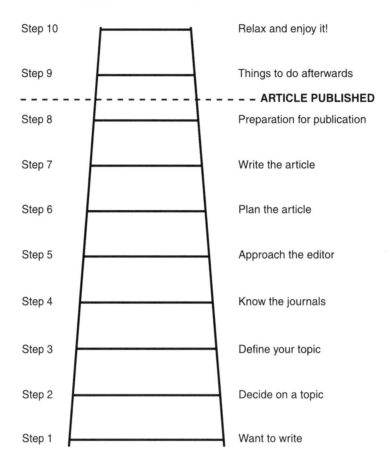

Step 10	Relax and enjoy it!
Step 9	Things to do afterwards
	ARTICLE PUBLISHED
Step 8	Preparation for publication
Step 7	Write the article
Step 6	Plan the article
Step 5	Approach the editor
Step 4	Know the journals
Step 3	Define your topic
Step 2	Decide on a topic
Step 1	Want to write

Figure 1.1 The 'writing ladder'.

In this chapter we shall look at ways of defining your topic and refining it to suit the audience you have in mind, as an essential step towards acceptance and publication.

☞ **Rushing into writing without defining your topic rarely saves time in the long term!**

What if you know that you want to write, but you don't know what to write about? In this case, you are poised on step 1 of the writing ladder. You may be in this situation if:

- you have already had one or more articles published, and you are now hooked on the fame/money/ego trip/academic merry-go-round, so you are desperate to keep publishing
- you think that there may be fame/money/credibility in being published, so you want to start writing
- your Trust, manager or course leader expects you to write 'something for the journals', so you feel obliged to do so.

In this case, you need to have some general ideas which you can then refine using the process described below. Later in this chapter we shall consider how to generate specific ideas from everyday practice.

DEFINING YOUR PARTICULAR TOPIC

We shall start from the point where you know what you want to write about, since this is probably the most common situation for which nurses seek advice. Your topic may be:

- a project you have been involved in
- an award you have received
- a clinical condition or case in which you are particularly interested
- a new development in the treatment or management of people in your clinical area
- an opinion you would like to express about a clinical, professional or employment topic.

There are three key questions to ask about your topic, which are shown in Box 2.1. Some general answers are listed in Box 2.2, to illustrate some of the options. These need to be refined and focused if they are to help in the next stages of preparing the article. Box 2.3 shows my five most recent articles, defined using the three key questions.

It may take a while for you to be sure what you want to write, for whom and why. Take as long as necessary to decide, and don't be afraid to change your mind – until you are sure what you want to write, you will not be able to explain it to anybody else!

Box 2.1:   **Three key questions to ask about a topic**

- What am I writing about?
- Who am I writing it for?
- Why am I telling them this?

Box 2.2:   Examples of general answers to the key questions

What?	Who for?	Why?
New development	Surgical nurses	Give information
Basic knowledge	Nursing students	Provide blueprint
Topical issue	Midwives in SCBUs*	Entertain
Significant event	Practice nurses	Start debate
Professional issue	Nurse executives	Highlight problem
Personal opinion	Male nurses	Spread good practice
Project	Health visitors	Publicise research
Personal experience	All nurses**	Contribute to knowledge

---

*Special Care Baby Units

**'All nurses' is not usually a helpful category for clinical articles. Few clinical topics are likely to be relevant to all nurses, and it makes the article much more difficult to plan and write, since you cannot know what level of previous knowledge and experience 'all nurses' have. However, some professional issues (e.g. patient advocacy) and general issues (e.g. prevention of violence against nurses) may be relevant across a broad spectrum of nurses.

Box 2.3:   Five recent articles defined using the three key questions

Topic	Target readership	Purpose	Journal/magazine
Recent publicity about nurses	General nurses	Entertain	*Nursing Standard*
Clinical governance	Practice nurses	Inform	*Practice Nurse*
Clinical governance	GPs and audit facilitators	Inform	*Audit Trends*
Primary care groups	GPs	Entertain	*Doctor*
Organisational development and primary care groups	Nurse managers	Inform/debate	*Nursing Management*

To experiment with the process, let us take the example given above, of the topic 'our new day-case unit'.

- *'What am I writing about?'* Our new day-case unit.
- *'Who am I writing it for?'* Other nurses on surgical day-case units.

- *'Why am I telling them this?'* Because our unit is really good and could be an example to them all.

This has started the process of defining the topic, but has not yet taken it far enough. An editor might ask, 'What about your new unit? Day-case units aren't new, so what is different about yours? Why would other nurses on day-case units want to read about yours?' (Note here that the editor, as well as carrying out his or her own job of commissioning suitable articles for the journal, is also acting as unpaid advisor to the author, since these are exactly the questions you need to ask yourself before you can plan and write your article.)

You need to use the same questions again to focus more narrowly on specific aspects of the topic.

- *'What am I writing about...exactly?'* The patient-centred, multidisciplinary team approach to gynaecological cases on our day-case unit.
- *'Who am I writing it for...precisely?'* Nurses and managers on both day-case and in-patient wards which admit patients for gynaecological procedures. (Because our approach could be adapted to either kind of ward, but focuses on women needing gynaecological surgery, it could not be directly applied to a general surgery unit.)
- *'Why am I telling them this...really?'* To share information about practice which has been shown to be effective and popular with patients, so that other units could introduce similar practice if it was appropriate to them.

Box 2.4 demonstrates how the general topic of 'our day-case unit' has been defined by answering these three questions. The information discovered through this process can be used in several ways. Focusing on the topic of the article through the use of the three key questions has:

- started to define the content of the article (*multidisciplinary teamwork and patient-centred approach for gynaecological surgery*), which will help with planning the article, finding what is relevant to include and what should be left out, and the kind of research for references which might be required
- clarified who it is aimed at (*surgical nurses and managers of units where gynaecological surgery is carried out*), which will help with targeting a journal with an appropriate readership
- identified the purpose of the article (*to give information and a 'blueprint' for others to follow*), which will help to decide the style as well as the content of the article, and to suggest which journal it should be targeted towards.

☞ **Always answer all three questions. Just deciding on the exact topic will not prepare you for effective planning, writing and targeting of the article.**

Some possible answers to the three questions as well as the routing towards

Box 2.4:   A topic defined: 'our day-case unit'

What is the topic?
The innovative way in which different disciplines within the team share the care of women attending for gynaecological operations, so that the woman feels in control of the process and can exercise some degree of choice

Who is it being written for?
Nurses on day units or in-patient wards dealing with gynaecological patients, as the way of working could probably be adapted to either setting. Also for nurse managers of such units, who might want to try out this way of working. Could also be of interest to nurses on surgical units dealing with other kinds of surgery, as the principles could be adapted to any group of patients

Why?
To share good practice, and to give nurses in other areas a 'blueprint' to copy or adapt as appropriate

---

Box 2.5:   Why you need to answer all three questions

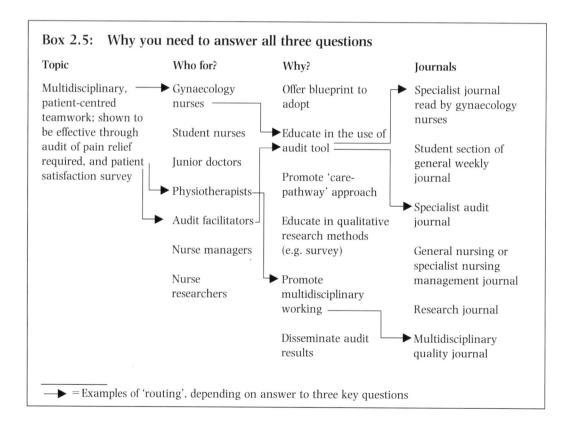

Topic	Who for?	Why?	Journals
Multidisciplinary, patient-centred teamwork; shown to be effective through audit of pain relief required, and patient satisfaction survey	Gynaecology nurses	Offer blueprint to adopt	Specialist journal read by gynaecology nurses
	Student nurses	Educate in the use of audit tool	Student section of general weekly journal
	Junior doctors	Promote 'care-pathway' approach	
	Physiotherapists		Specialist audit journal
	Audit facilitators	Educate in qualitative research methods (e.g. survey)	General nursing or specialist nursing management journal
	Nurse managers		
	Nurse researchers	Promote multidisciplinary working	Research journal
		Disseminate audit results	Multidisciplinary quality journal

⟶ = Examples of 'routing', depending on answer to three key questions appropriate types of journals are shown in Box 2.5, to demonstrate the importance of taking all three questions into account.

☞ **It is essential to be as specific as possible in relation to your particular topic when answering the three key questions!**

Take another example from those listed above, namely the 'aromatherapy in labour' topic. The answer to the question 'what am I writing about?' could be:

● my research demonstrating the effectiveness of aromatherapy for pain relief in the first stage of labour
● a review of all the published research on the effectiveness of aromatherapy for pain relief in labour
● my experience, both as a mother and as a midwife, of trying to use aromatherapy for pain relief in my own labour, and the opposition encountered
● the difference between medical and midwifery staff's attitudes to complementary medicines in the labour suite
● our unit's standard-setting process for the use of complementary therapies
● a survey of all maternity units in the North-West region with regard to their attitudes to and protocols for the use of aromatherapy in labour.

There are many more possible topics which could be included under the heading of 'aromatherapy in labour', so clearly such a general heading is not going to help an editor to decide whether he or she is interested in your article, nor will it help you to look for reference materials, to plan the structure of your article or to decide which journal to write it for. Defining the topic further, as in the list above, begins to deal with the first of the three key questions. Then you need to ask two questions: 'who am I writing this for?' and 'why am I telling them this?'. The various possible answers to all three questions will direct you both towards the type and style of article you are writing, and suitable journals (*see* Box 2.6 for the rest of the aromatherapy example).

WRITE AS YOU READ 2.1

☞ Answer the three key questions for the topic you have in mind.

Box 2.6: A topic defined: aromatherapy in labour		
Topic	**Who for?**	**Why?**
My experience of trying to use aromatherapy for pain relief in first-stage labour	Midwives in labour suites	To highlight a problem area of practice

This is the kind of exercise which you could do in your head, during a train journey, over the ironing or while on a long walk. However, it is sometimes easier to be clear with yourself if you write down your decisions. Write the general topic at the top of the page, and then divide the page roughly into three, and answer each question, as shown in Box 2.7 (you could photocopy this box and use it as a template).

By doing this all on one page, you can easily check each answer against the other, to make sure that your decisions are logical and the end result makes sense. For example, the decision to write about the ethical dilemmas which nurses face, for a readership of medical researchers, in order to entertain them, is not a logical one!

At the end of the process, you should be able to condense your decisions into a single sentence suitable for the ears of a busy editor. For example, 'I'm thinking of writing an article about the new CFC-free inhalers in asthma treatment, for practice nurses who run asthma clinics, to update them'. There will be more detail to discuss (*see* Chapter 4), but at least you will be presenting a clear and attractive proposition in your first sentence. Put this summary sentence in a box at the bottom of the page – it helps to have it in front of you at every stage between this important decision and publication!

When you have defined the topic of your article, who it is aimed at, and your purpose in writing it, you are ready to start looking for a suitable journal to approach with your idea. This is discussed in detail in the next chapter.

LOOKING FOR A TOPIC

It is possible, however, that you do not have even a general topic in mind. In this case you are at step 1 on the writing ladder, knowing that you want to write, but not knowing what to write about. In this case, start with the 'why?' question – not 'why are you writing this for that audience?' (that will come later) but 'why are you writing at all?'

- Is it to get your name in the journals for your own satisfaction? If so, you have a very wide range of possibilities open to you, and you are going to have a lot of fun!
- Is it to satisfy the demands of a course leader or manager, who wants you to write 'something' so that you can claim to have been published? In this case, your topic needs to be appropriate to the course or to your job, and the field of possibilities is beginning to narrow.
- Is it to satisfy the demand of a manager or colleagues that you 'write up' a particular project or enterprise? In this case your topic is largely determined for you, and you only have to decide which aspect of it to focus on. You can go directly to Box 2.7 and start to define your topic.

If you are writing for a course, or because it is expected in your job, then you need to

Box 2.7:   Defining your own topic

General topic:

What am I writing about. . .exactly?

Who am I writing this for. . .precisely?

Why exactly am I telling them this?

SUMMARY:

look around within those areas for a topic. Suppose your course is on 'Family Planning in Society'. Possible topics for an article could include:

- technical issues (methods of contraception, physiology of the female reproductive system, etc.)
- professional issues (nurse-prescribing issues in family planning, clinical supervision for clinic nurses, issues of confidentiality in young people's clinics, etc.)
- quality-oriented issues (audit of clinics against national guidelines, patient satisfaction surveys, debate about appropriate training, etc.)
- opinion/experience (how it felt to work with 12 to 14-years-olds, the Case of the Missing Coil, etc.).

Once you start looking for a topic to write about, you are bound to find one. There is no area of practice or experience which could not furnish material for an article.

👉 **Remember that an article does not have to be about something new or particularly significant** (*see* Chapter 1).

Once you have decided on a topic, you can move to Box 2.7 as well, to define exactly what you are writing about, for whom, and why.

If you are in this second category, of writing to satisfy someone else's demands, it would be worth checking your idea for an article with them, once you have decided on your summary sentence, but before you go any further with the process. If they are not happy with the topic, you may want to save yourself the trouble of working through the later stages of preparation. Or, of course, you may decide that you have worked up a very good idea, and you are going to pursue it in any case.

For those in the first category, who 'want to write because they want to write', the fun starts here! There are many different forms of writing you can choose apart from the traditional article. Start with the 'why?' question from the original three key questions. Why are you writing this? To educate, amuse, disseminate, explain or debate? Then choose a form you would like to try which is suited to your purpose (*see* Box 2.8). Identifying and refining your topic, in this situation, comes last.

Suppose, for example, that you have decided you want to devise an educational clinical quiz. You might decide to aim it at nurses on metabolic units, because you work on one, and your colleagues seem to like that kind of thing. Your topic needs to be clinical, and related to metabolic disease. It also needs to provide a reasonable number of questions which have unequivocal answers, so that the multiple-choice format will work. You will now be able to identify some suitable and specific topics – perhaps diabetes mellitus or (to be more interesting) diabetes insipidus. To decide on the level of difficulty of the questions, you will then need to ask yourself, 'Who am I writing this for?'

In this situation, you are taking the key questions in a different order to someone who starts with an idea for a topic. Instead of asking 'What? Who for? Why?', you are asking 'Why? What? Who for?' Provided that all three questions are addressed

Box 2.8:   Forms for functions

Function	Possible forms
To entertain	Quiz Humorous narrative Satirical column Feature Cartoon Opinion piece
To educate	Article with assessment Research report Descriptive feature Quiz Letter Literature review Project report
To start/contribute to debate	Opinion piece Letter Descriptive feature
To analyse policy	Opinion piece Feature Research report
To disseminate good practice	Project report Audit report Research report Descriptive feature Literature review

before you try to identify a suitable journal or approach an editor, this does not matter at all.

To take one more example before you tackle your own, suppose you want to write a piece solely in order to amuse and entertain readers. To decide what the topic will be, you could:

- think of an incident at work which could be recounted entertainingly (I had an article published in the *American Journal of Nursing* based on my experiences of carrying out a health check on a 90-year-old woman who was fitter and more active than I was)

- browse through a dictionary of medical quotations or other relevant books to find something you could build an article on (I wrote an article for the *Nursing Standard*, which was subsequently reprinted in the *Guardian*, based on an old public health report about people dying of 'distraction', 'evil' and 'surfeit')
- check lists of anniversaries, commemorations and special 'health-topic days' for ideas (I have already done 'Diarrhoea Day', but there must be some mileage to be had from the anniversary of the invention of the electric wheelchair, for example)
- watch the news for snippets which could be turned into humorous pieces (such as the discovery of viruses on Mars).

Once you have an idea, think about who you will be writing the article for – and you have started to answer the three key questions in Box 2.7. Refine your topic, fill in the summary sentence, and you will be ready for the next chapter, on finding a suitable outlet for your article.

SUMMARY

Much delay and irritation later in the process can be prevented if you take time at the beginning to be clear about what you are writing about, for whom and why. Preparing a brief statement summarising your decision will help you to find the right journal for your article, and to sell your idea to an editor, as well as to plan and write the article itself.

CHAPTER THREE

KNOWING YOUR
JOURNALS

You've got to really read the journal you want to get published in first – lots of authors obviously don't read the journal, then they write things at the wrong level, or pick on subjects we've already covered a lot.

(Judith Podmore, 'Nursing Management')

If you have worked through the first two chapters of this workbook, then you will have decided on a topic for an article, and defined exactly what you are going to write about, the target readership, and the purpose of writing it. So why stop now to think about the journals, rather than get on with writing the article? The simplest and best reason is that:

☛ **Knowing the journals vastly increases your chances of getting published.**

Personally, I would rate the formatting and targeting of an article to a particular journal as the most important factor in successful writing for publication, and you cannot tailor your article to a particular publication unless you know it well. On the few occasions in recent years when I have had articles rejected, the reason has been that I did not bother to check out the journal before sending in the article. Suitably embarrassed and ashamed, I then had to search for an appropriate journal, approach the editor, and revise and rewrite the article to fit the new journal's requirements. It serves me right for ignoring my own number one rule!

It is absolutely essential to get to know the journals in the market-place for articles, because:

- rejection is terribly demoralising
- nothing damages your credibility with the journal's editor and staff faster than submitting material that is clearly unsuitable

- rejection wastes time, not only in terms of the months you may spend waiting to receive the rejection letter, but also in rewriting and resubmitting the article.

So how do you get to know the journals, magazines and other publications (these names will be used interchangeably in this chapter)?

FINDING THE JOURNALS

If you have a specific article in mind, you are really only interested in the range of publications which might be possible markets for that article. However, do not fall into the trap of only considering the one or two journals which you personally read. They may be very familiar, and seem to be appropriate, but such a restriction would unnecessarily limit your opportunities to be published. Aim to look at a minimum of four or five journals as a start, so that you have a clearer view of the choices that are open to you. There are several easy ways to find some journals to look at with an eye to publication.

- Scan the journal shelves of the local nursing library, hospital or health-centre library. Go for the 'current issues' shelves rather than back numbers (*see* Box 3.1).
- Look at the listings of journals held at the library. I guarantee that they will include numerous specialist journals that you never even dreamed existed (*see* Box 3.2)!
- Check among the target audience. If your article is aimed at midwives, ask some midwives what they read, or nip into their unit and see what journals are kept on the wards.

Box 3.1:   A word of warning

Always look at the most recent issues of a publication, as editors, sections, format and approach change regularly. It is easy to be caught out by looking at an old copy of a journal.

Box 3.2:   Some journals you never knew existed

- *Journal of Human Lactation*
- *Computers in Nursing*
- *Diabetic Foot*

☞ **Take the broadest possible perspective on your article, in order to give yourself the widest possible scope for publication (*see* Box 3.3).**

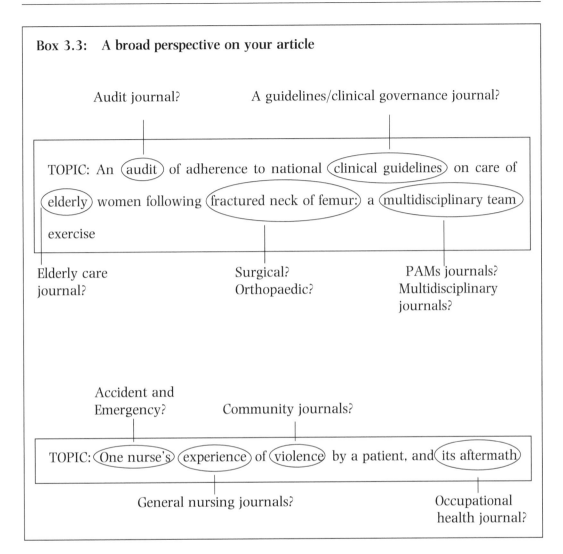

Box 3.3:   A broad perspective on your article

Audit journal?   A guidelines/clinical governance journal?

TOPIC: An audit of adherence to national clinical guidelines on care of elderly women following fractured neck of femur: a multidisciplinary team exercise

Elderly care
journal?   Surgical?   PAMs journals?
                                  Orthopaedic?   Multidisciplinary
                                                            journals?

Accident and
Emergency?   Community journals?

TOPIC: One nurse's experience of violence by a patient, and its aftermath

General nursing journals?   Occupational
                                             health journal?

ASSESSING THE JOURNALS

Once you have found a handful of journals which look as if they might be suitable vehicles for conveying your article to its intended audience, you will need to assess them. The best way to do this is to take the two or three most recent issues and explore them systematically. This need only take a few minutes per journal (you could copy and use Box 3.4 as a permanent record), and saves hours of wasted time.

The following key pieces of information should be extracted when assessing a journal.

- Who is it written for?
- Who is it written by?

Box 3.4: Journal assessment sheet

Journal name:

Editor:

Telephone numbers:

Aims:

Readership (stated/unstated):

Sections:

Recent content:

Guidelines for publication: in journal and copied/
                                        tel number to send for ....

- What type of articles does it publish?

☞ **It cannot be over-emphasised how important it is to look at the very latest issues when searching for this information.**

Editors, sections, aims, tone and content all change over time, and it is a waste of your time and credibility to tailor an article for a section that no longer exists, or ring up and ask for an editor who left 6 months ago!

ASSESSING THE TARGET READERSHIP OF THE JOURNAL

To do this, look first at the title. *'Surgical Nurse'* seems clear enough, but is the readership as broad as that, or does it focus on one type of surgery, or one setting (acute general hospitals)? *'Primary Health Care'* is a very broad title, but is the readership equally spread among all nurses in the community (including health visitors, community midwives and community psychiatric nurses), or is the journal really of interest only to district nurses and practice nurses?

Sometimes the targeted readership is stated on the cover, or inside the journal itself. For example:

- *Practice Nurse* has a line under the title which reads 'the journal for nurses in general practice'
- *Community Practitioner* is 'the journal of the Community Practitioners' and Health Visitors' Association'
- *Practice Manager* is 'the journal of professional management in general practice'.

If it is not explicitly stated, you can clarify the readership by looking further into the journal. Underneath the title, or on the contents page, you may find a 'mission statement' or aim. Some current examples are listed in Box 3.5. These statements are excellent guides both to readership (which may be mentioned specifically) and the type of articles which the journal is likely to accept. For example, *Primary Health Care Research and Development* describes itself as 'an outlet for the presentation of research findings which are directly applicable to practice, as well as a forum for researchers and practitioners to debate issues and exchange information'. Clearly this journal should welcome approaches about research reports, or practitioner pieces on the experience of implementing research findings, but it is unlikely to be a vehicle for satirical political comment or clinical quizzes!

Another way to assess the target readership of the journal is to look down the contents list and note:

- the sections into which the journal is divided
- the content of individual articles.

Box 3.5:   Example of journal 'mission statements'

'*Nursing Times* is the independent voice of nursing. It is radical, challenging and professional, and aims to inform, inspire and entertain. It campaigns for a better deal for patients and for the nurses, midwives and health visitors who care for them'

The *Journal of Clinical Nursing* aims 'to help nursing, midwifery and health visiting practitioners to gain an up-to-date, evidence-based knowledge relevant in their clinical practice'

'*NT Research* will...value formal, well-tested expertise in nursing research and make it accessible to practitioners. It will:

• publish original research on nursing topics and themes
• process material efficiently
• disseminate research with the aim of encouraging evidence-based practice and improving the quality of patient care
• provide a safe, educationally sound environment for authors to develop their research and writing skills and participate in peer review'

The *British Journal of Community Nursing*: 'promoting excellence in primary care'

The sections tell you not only what types of articles might be welcome, but how much of the journal is devoted to each kind of article. For example, *Nursing Standard* currently has the following sections:

• news
• analysis
• features
• perspectives
• art and science
• career development.

Of these sections, 'perspectives' has the most articles – double the number in the art and science section – so there is plenty of scope for opinion pieces, debates, letters and responses to topical issues. There is no section on primary research reports, so this is probably not the journal for that 5000-word article on your Masters research.

Similarly, a review of the content of the articles which have recently been published is a very good guide to the readership of the journal, and the kind of articles the editor might be looking for. A journal may claim to be for 'all community nurses', but if the contents of the last three issues are all about mental health, care of the elderly, changes in social policy and research into ageing, it is unlikely to have a large readership among community paediatric nurses.

Having assessed the target readership of the journals you have chosen, you will know whether you can reach the target audience for your article through any of these publications. If so, you can move on to the next stage of the assessment.

WHO IS WRITING IN THE JOURNAL?

The editorial page of the journal usually includes a box containing the names of the people who work on the journal. Note the name of the editor, and of the editors of sections to which you might want to contribute, in preparation for the time when you contact them, and later submit your article. The journal's telephone number will also be on this page.

☞ **This is the time when you should really be looking at the very latest issue. Journal staff seem to move on very quickly!**

Now look through the journal and note who has written the articles and columns that it features. Names appear at the beginning of the article of course, but there is often additional information at the end, or in a side panel, giving the author's 'day job' and qualifications. You will usually find articles by:

- practising nurses
- freelance writers
- members of other professions (e.g. doctors)
- people with specialist skills in a particular area (e.g. dietitians).

Box 3.6 lists some of the articles in the current issues of *Nursing Times*, and the information given about their authors, as an example.

The fact that these different types of author are published indicates the opportunities available. As a practising nurse, you have credibility and clinical knowledge, and many journals would be keen to use this. If you are not currently working as a nurse, you can always write as a freelancer, and clearly there is scope for freelancers in most of the journals. As a nurse, you are not restricted to writing for the nursing journals. If doctors, dietitians and counsellors can write for nursing journals, using their specialist knowledge and experience, then nurses can also write for medical, therapy and other publications, provided that they assess the journal thoroughly and tailor their material appropriately.

☞ **Do not be put off if the authors in a journal all seem to have a string of letters after their name, or have high-flying jobs. Their articles are not generally accepted because of who they are, but because of what they have to say, and your article will be judged in the same way.**

Box 3.6:   Some articles and authors – *Nursing Times*

Topic	Author
Patient attitudes (comment/ opinion)	Nurse inspector, health authority
Induction for new nurses (comment)	Staff nurse, neurology day care, children's hospital
Day-case surgery for ligament reconstruction (description/ example)	Operations manager, day-surgery unit
Education for day surgery (description/comment)	Senior lecturer, university school of health
Alcoholism and drug dependency (personal experience)	Counsellor
Removal of sutures (clinical/ educational)	Staff nurse, cardiology; infection control nurse; professional development nurse
Internet libraries (information)	Lecturer, university
Asian people and mental health problems (survey report/ example)	Transcultural nurses
Mental Health Act powers (information)	Nurse/solicitor
Link between stress and cancer (evidence review)	Research fellow, university

---

WHAT SORT OF ARTICLES DOES THE JOURNAL PUBLISH?

You have already scanned the contents list for clues about the usual readership of the journal you are assessing. Note also the different kinds of articles which the journal publishes. They may include clinical articles, comments, book reviews, project reports and literature reviews, among others. Even the most 'serious' and academic journals have some pages devoted to material other than lengthy research reports, to provide some variety for the reader. For example, the *Journal of Clinical Nursing* may contain up to 10 long articles (2000–5000 words) in each issue, but also carries 'Research in brief' (500 words) and literature reviews.

As well as the content of the articles, look at the approaches used. They may be:

- narrative, telling the reader about the topic, incident or project
- personal opinion (written in the first person)
- commentary on a current issue (but not written in the first person)
- reporting of a research study, including an objective analysis of the methodological strengths and weaknesses of the study, and a discussion of the conclusions drawn from it
- reporting of a case, project or event, combining narrative with some commentary
- educational, sometimes including tasks or exercises for the reader to complete, and even (in the case of the Royal College of Nursing continuing education articles) a multiple-choice assessment paper.

Knowing what kind of approach is used in articles in the journal you are considering is important in choosing which publication to target. If *Diabetic Medicine* reaches the readers you want to target, and publishes on topics similar to yours, you might still need to discard it as a possible market if you do not feel that you could write in the objective and rigorously referenced style it uses. Similarly, if you want to write an opinion or debate piece, check that the journal uses articles with that approach.

Incidentally, when you are an established writer with a long and successful publication pedigree, you may suggest to an editor that they might like to introduce a new approach or feature to their journal (e.g. humour in a research journal, or distance-learning articles in a practitioner magazine). The editor might just take you up on the idea. However, if you are an inexperienced writer, such a suggestion is likely to look like laziness (you can't be bothered to find a suitable publication, so you expect this one to change to accommodate what you want to write). Avoid this strategy for now.

Once you have assessed the journals for their readership, authors and typical content, you are ready to identify which of them you will target for your article.

➤ **Once you have narrowed your choice to one or two journals, find and photocopy their Guidelines for Contributors page or box. This will be a very important guide to the planning of your article.**

If the guidelines are not published in the journal, there is usually a telephone number to contact in order to obtain a copy.

There is one more assessment which you need to make before moving on to the next step of the writing ladder – approaching the editor – which is to check what your chosen journal has published recently on your topic, or on related topics.

☞ **Don't despair if your topic seems to have been covered recently in your chosen publication.**

If the recently published article has covered exactly the same ground, using the same approach, you will find it difficult to persuade the editor to look at your article. Indeed to offer such a similar article would suggest to the editor that you have not bothered to read the journal, but have chosen it at random. This is unlikely to elicit a positive or encouraging response! You might need to choose a different journal to approach.

However, even if the general topic has been covered, your particular angle on the topic may still be acceptable. For example, the *Journal of Substance Misuse* may have had many articles on the topic of solvent abuse, but if you are writing about a novel approach to educating children about the dangers of glue sniffing, you have every chance of engaging the editor's interest. If your topic is a common one (e.g. the use of antibiotics), start to think about the things that make your proposed article different. Perhaps:

- it takes a humorous approach to a previously pedestrian subject
- you will write it from a nursing rather than the usual medical perspective
- you have personal experience to draw on and add interest to the article
- your audit of prescribing involved patients' views for the first time
- the research you describe has some radically different results from other studies.

There will be more on ways to make your article irresistible to the editor in the next chapter.

SUMMARY

Knowing your journals means deliberately assessing a range of publications to find out their target readership, what sort of authors write for them, and what types of article they usually publish. It allows you to make an informed and effective choice of a journal whose editor you will approach with your article idea. If you do not check out the journals in this way before you write, you greatly increase the likelihood of your article being rejected because:

- the journal does not publish the type of article you have written
- the style and approach of your article do not fit the journal's style
- the topic of your article will not be of interest to the journal's readers
- the journal has just published something very similar.

WRITE AS YOU READ 3.1

☞ Now decide which journal you are going to approach with your article idea.

Visit your local nursing library, and select five or six journals which might be suitable for your article. Remember that they need not necessarily be nursing journals. Then make some photocopies of Box 3.4, and use it to record your assessment of the latest two or three issues of the journals you have chosen. Remember that you are particularly interested in:

- the target readership of the journal
- the types of article that are published.

When you have finished the assessment, you should have:

- a definite publication in mind to approach with your article idea
- a note of the editor's (and section editors') name and telephone numbers
- notes on the journal's aims, target readership, sections and typical content
- a copy of the journal's Guidelines for Contributors, or the number to ring to obtain them.

When you have all of this information, you are ready to talk to the editor about your article.

CHAPTER FOUR

APPROACHING AN EDITOR

Most editors are happy to be rung up. It's better if the author rings early on, before they have an article ready – then the editor can say, 'focus on this aspect' or 'this is what we need'. People tend to ring too late on.

(Judith Podmore, 'Nursing Management')

On the phone, try to be brief, concise and friendly – even if the editor appears to be a grouchy old sod.

(Daniel Allen, 'Mental Health Nursing')

The idea of ringing up the editor of a journal to talk about your article before you have written it may fill you with horror, or simply incomprehension. Why should you put yourself through that, when you already know exactly what you are going to write about, and you have the journal's Guidelines for Contributors in front of you?

Many nurses don't make contact with the journal before writing, and many of them have their articles published. However, if your aim is to maximise your chances of publication, you are much more likely to succeed if you talk to the editor first.

WHAT THE EDITOR CAN TELL YOU

If you have a copy of the Guidelines for Contributors, and you have researched the latest issues of the journal to see what topics have been covered recently, you may wonder what else the editor can tell you. The answer is that they may be able to tell you several very important things:

- *what articles they already have on their desks* – if they already have an article on your proposed topic of electronic fetal monitoring during the first stage of labour, they are unlikely to want another in the near future. In this case you can save yourself the time and trouble of writing the article and take your excellent idea elsewhere

☞ **In this case, making contact with the editor will probably save you at least 6 months (2–3 months of writing, and 3 months of waiting for the rejection letter).**

- *what articles they have commissioned* – that is, articles which they have asked someone to write for them, and which should be on the way. There is some hope here, even if the topic is identical to yours. The commissioned author may not deliver, or the manuscript may not be up to scratch, or you may be able to persuade the editor that they need a second perspective (i.e. yours) on the same topic. If not, you still have the opportunity to let them know that you are another experienced midwife who is willing and able to write for publication – an opportunity you would not have had if you had simply sent in an article which was quickly rejected because they were waiting for the commissioned one
- *what types of topics, features or series they are planning for the future* – many journals plan well in advance, and may have a year's worth of topics mapped out, but without authors' names attached. Your telephone call gives the editor a chance to shape your idea to fit in with his or her plans.

☞ **This gives you the chance to write the article that the editor wants to print, rather than the one you want to write, and saves you spending time, 6 months down the line turning the latter into the former!**

None of this vital information can be found by looking at recent issues of the journal – you need to go 'in house' to find it. Therefore, daunting as it might seem at first, it really is a good idea to talk to the editor of your chosen journal before you even begin to write your article.

☞ **I have tried writing instead of telephoning. I have never had a reply to a written contact, even when the letter was faxed.**

PREPARATION

Editors are used to being telephoned by authors and potential contributors, and appreciate the opportunity to refine and tailor an idea to suit their needs – it is, after all, entirely in their best interests! In my experience they are usually patient, receptive and very helpful. There has only ever been one editor whom I found consistently intimidating, but I did succeed in getting four articles into his publication, and a tidy sum of money for doing so, so I coped with the trauma of ringing him!

However, as you would expect, editors are very busy people, and the more prepared, logical and professional you can be in presenting your idea, the better for all concerned.

☞ Never ring an editor on the spur of the moment with an unresearched idea. You are likely to make yourself feel silly and damage your credibility with the editor.

The key to a successful and professional conversation with an editor is preparation. You need to have to hand:

- your proposal
- the correct editor's contact details
- notes of the information you need to get from the editor
- pen and paper to note down what you agree to do.

YOUR PROPOSAL

This consists of five elements, three of which you already have. They are:

- your exact topic
- your target audience
- the purpose of writing.

This is information you decided on and refined in the course of the last two chapters. The other two elements are the answers to two questions that the editor may well ask.

- Why you?
- Why now?

The editor is unlikely to say baldly, 'And why should I want this article from you?' However, to preserve the reputation of the journal, he or she is going to want to be sure that the clinical or professional articles published in it are topical, relevant and factually accurate, as well as interesting and acceptable to the journal's readership. This does not mean that you have to be at the top of your branch of the profession. You may be the right person to write this article because:

- you are a clinical specialist ('expert') in the topic (e.g. a diabetes specialist nurse writing about insulin-delivery devices)
- you have a lot of experience in the area (e.g. a practice nurse with 10 years of experience writing about patient expectations in general practice)
- you designed/led/evaluated the project (i.e. this is a piece of work you know well)

- your job is to deal with this issue (e.g. a ward manager writing about staff support, or a university lecturer writing an educational article)
- you have the expertise or experience to research the topic and present it in a suitable form for the journal (e.g. you are a teacher, or an experienced writer).

The situation is slightly different for opinion pieces or humorous pieces, as opposed to clinical or professional articles. In this case, what you do as a job, or where your years of experience lie, is less relevant than whether you can express yourself clearly and/or humorously. However, you should be prepared to be asked what you do and where you work. It may help that you are a nurse, if you are targeting a nursing journal, as opinion and comment carry much more weight if they come from within rather than outside the profession.

Describing who you are, and therefore why you should be the one to write the article, may involve more than one reason. You could be writing about precipitate labour as a midwife, or as a midwife who has had an unusual amount of experience of such labours, or as a midwife who has had such a labour herself. The editor may be particularly attracted by a new 'twist' to a familiar topic – perhaps an article on the role of the health visitor in running women's groups, written by a male health visitor, or an article on managing post-operative pain, written by a surgical nurse who is also a qualified aromatherapist.

☞ **Don't be shy about promoting yourself as author of your article. Unless your topic is very unusual, there will be many people who could write something similar, and you need to convince the editor that they want *you* to write it.**

The fifth element – the answer to the question 'Why now?' – gives you another opportunity to make a wavering editor want your article. If you can convince the editor that your article is particularly topical, and that your topic is one that nurses most want (or need) to read about, then you greatly increase the chance of the editor at least asking to read it. There are plenty of ways in which you can do this.

- Link the topic to recent policy changes or trends (e.g. 'With the increase in very dependent patients being nursed at home, this is a good time to review the competencies needed by district nurses').
- Link it to proposed changes in the nursing profession (e.g. 'There is a lot of debate at the moment about the regulation of healthcare support workers, and the project I am describing shows how support workers can take on some very specialised roles under the supervision of a clinical nurse specialist').
- Relate it to recent articles in the journal (e.g. 'Your series about management has focused on different kinds of specialist units, but hasn't mentioned out-patients: my research project showed how the patient's experience in the out-patient department affects their perception of care in all parts of the hospital').
- Link the topic to an anniversary or significant date (e.g. 'Our unit opened 100

years ago this September: my article compares the experience of patients with sexually transmitted diseases last century with the treatments and prognosis today').

☞ **Remember all those articles around the 50th anniversary of the National Health Service? Some of us made a few pounds and some easy publications from that one!**

- For opinion or comment pieces, link the topic to recent events or previous contributions to the opinion pages (e.g. 'Last week you had a piece from a nurse defending euthanasia in special-care baby units: I'd like to put the other side of the story').

☞ **It is important to remember that 'topical' means different things on different time-scales.**

A weekly magazine will have a shorter 'lead time' (i.e. time from final deadline for contributions to publication) than a quarterly journal. Allowing time for writing the article, and the process of publication, you may need to think 6 months ahead. Ask yourself how topical your 'topical' article will be in 6 months' time. However, opinion pieces are often accepted and published on a time-scale of weeks, or even days, rather than months, so topicality is much more straightforward.

☞ **If you feel motivated to write an opinion piece on something in the news, or a recent article in the journal, you need to do it very quickly. If you wait for your days off the following week, you may well be too late.**

THE EDITOR'S DETAILS

In preparation for your telephone call, you need the name and telephone number of the relevant editor, taken from the front page of the *latest* issue of the journal. In some publications, you will only find the editor's and sub-editor's details, in which case you need to ring the editor, who makes the decisions about the journal's content. In others, such as the weekly nursing magazines, you will find the names of section editors (e.g. 'opinion editor', 'clinical editor', 'primary care editor' or 'continuing education editor'). Choose the section most suited to the type of article you are offering, and start with that editor, rather than the main journal editor. Section editors are usually easier to contact, and keen to find good articles for their section. Often they have been in clinical practice in the relevant area, and therefore understand the issues involved.

WHAT YOU NEED TO ASK THE EDITOR

It is useful to make a note of the information you want to obtain from the editor when they have agreed to look at your article, so that you don't forget in the heat of the moment. In particular, you will want to know:

- the word length required
- the deadline for delivery.

☞ **Make sure that you have read the journal's Guidelines for Contributors before you ring the editor, if these are printed in the journal. If they are not, it is quite acceptable to ask the editor for them, but if they are regularly printed in the journal, asking for them suggests that you have not even looked at the publication!**

The Guidelines for Contributors will probably tell you what word length is required for different types of article. It is still worth asking the editor for confirmation, as they may want to vary it. However, you don't need to check every detail of the guidelines with them. If the guidelines state 'articles must be typed or word processed on one side of A4, with text double spaced and wide margins all round', then this is how it must be presented, and there is no need to discuss the matter with the editor.

MAKING THE TELEPHONE CALL

It is essential to telephone the editor when you have your notes in front of you, time for the conversation, and uninterrupted use of the phone. However, it is very likely that the editor you want will not be available when you ring, and someone will take your number so that they can call you back. Be prepared for this eventuality, by having a time and telephone number to suggest which means that they won't call you in the middle of a baby clinic or ward round.

If they do not return your call within the next couple of days, it is worth trying again. The lack of response does not mean that they have already decided to reject your idea! They are probably just very busy getting the next issue of the journal out on time.

☞ **Remember, at this stage you are 'selling' your idea. You need to make the running, persevere in the face of setbacks, and believe in your product!**

Sooner or later, you will be able to talk to the editor, and you will need to be:

- clear about what you are offering and why
- concise in your description of your idea and your expertise
- confident that what you are offering is a good idea, and that you can write the article you are proposing
- professional in your approach to the job of producing an article for the journal.

☞ **Remind yourself that you and the editor are both professionals in your different fields. You are neither a supplicant at the altar of publication, nor a professional superstar condescending to share your expertise!**

The notes you have made in preparation for the conversation will help with all of these requirements. The time spent refining your topic and researching the journal pays dividends in maintaining your confidence at this stage.

☞ **Expect the editor to ask questions about your topic, to question its content and timing, and to have to be persuaded about its merits. You will have to sell!**

So how might the conversation proceed? It is unlikely to take the form shown in Box 4.1. An editor would be taking a great risk to commission articles on this basis! As a more realistic example, Box 4.2 shows a summary of a conversation I had with a journal editor about two articles on reflective practice. This resulted in a commission for the articles (see Box 4.3 for the difference between accepting an idea and commissioning an article).

Box 4.1:   An unlikely conversation with an editor

Author: Hello, I'd like to write an article on testicular cancer for *Nurses Weekly*.
Editor: Great. What are you planning to cover?
Author: Oh, everything really.
Editor: Okay. So, can you give me 3000 words by, say, next Easter?
Author: Actually, I'm going to be away for most of February. How about next Summer?
Editor: Fine. It can go in the New Year issue, in our Men's Health supplement. Thanks for thinking of us.

You will see from Box 4.2 that there was much negotiation in that conversation with the editor. We negotiated about the topic (whether it was still of interest to practice nurses), what approach I would take (theoretical or practical), whether it needed to be one article or two, and when the articles could be submitted.

I had been intending to be fairly theoretical, thinking that this might be helpful for practice nurses undertaking specialist practitioner courses, but the editor was clearly wanting a much more practical approach, so I changed my plan. However, I held firm on the number of articles, feeling sure that I could not cover the topic adequately in one.

It is worth noting that I have written many articles for this journal, and I know the editor well. A writer offering a first article to this publication might not be able to hold out for two articles, if their writing and reliability is an unknown quantity. They would almost certainly not be offered a commission, but would probably be asked to send in their article 'on spec'.

Box 4.2:   Summary of my conversation with an editor about 'reflective practice' articles

RC: I wondered if you would be interested in two articles describing reflective practice for practice nurses?

Editor: I think we may have done reflective practice before – its been around for a while.

RC: Yes, but many more practice nurses are doing academic courses now, and keeping reflective diaries is a large part of most courses.

Editor: What would you include in it?

RC   I thought one article would be about the theoretical basis for reflective practice, and the other would describe the model they use in the Burford Nursing Development Unit, which could be easily applied to practice nursing.

Editor: I don't think we want too much emphasis on theory. We would need some practical examples from practice nursing.

RC: Yes, I could use practice nursing scenarios and examples, showing how the model would apply.

Editor: Couldn't you do it in one article?

RC: I really don't think there would be space to give some background, and describe the model, and then apply it, with examples, in one article.

Editor: Okay. But we would need practical examples in both articles, not just theory in the first.

RC: Right. How long would you want each article to be?

Editor: Between 1500 and 2000 words each.

RC: And when would you want the first?

Editor: What about 3 January for the first, and 3 February for the second?

THE OUTCOME

There are two possible outcomes to the 'selling' part of the conversation. The editor may agree to look at the article, or they may reject the idea as unsuitable for their journal.

If the editor does not accept the idea, and is not interested in seeing the article, you need to finish the conversation professionally and politely. 'Blow you, then, I'll offer it to *Nursing Times*!' (or similar) is not a good ending to the conversation. Thank them for their time, and exit gracefully. You may want to offer them another article in future, and your name is known and your reputation is founded solely on the telephone conversations you have had with them, so it is important to make a good impression for next time!

Box 4.3:   The difference between 'accepting an idea' and 'commissioning' an article

Accepting an idea	This is the most common editorial response, especially if you have not written much for the journal before. It means that the editor is happy to look at your article, but does not guarantee acceptance. You may be asked to revise your article after submission, or it may be rejected for a variety of reasons. Although it is not binding on you, failure to submit the article would damage your credibility with the editor and the journal.
Commissioning an article	This is a much more definite process. The editor will follow up the conversation with a commissioning letter, and will expect to receive your article on time and to specification. They will have pencilled the article into their plan for a particular issue, and failure to submit the article, although it will probably not lead you to court for breach of contract, will seriously damage your reputation.

☞ **Remember, the fact that this journal does not want your article at this time does not mean that no other journal will want it, or that it is inherently a bad idea (*see the Myths and Hard Facts in Chapter 1!*).**

The happier outcome is that the editor expresses an interest in seeing the article based on your idea. Now you need to do the following.

Agree the content

The editor may have ideas of their own about what they want to include or exclude from your article. As they know what else is coming up in the journal, it is usually wise to accept their suggestions. For example, they may say, 'We're about to do a series on alternative therapies, so can you leave that bit out, but say more about the new drugs for multiple sclerosis?' The answer to this should usually be 'yes'. However, if the whole point of your article was to describe the use of alternative therapies in treating MS, then either you have not described your idea very well, or the editor is being particularly difficult! You will need to decide whether you are willing to change your article fundamentally, or whether you would rather try a different journal with your original idea.

Check word length

The Guidelines for Contributors will have given some parameters, but the editor may want to vary these.

Agree the deadline for submission

The editor may suggest an alarmingly short deadline, because your article would fit well into a planned series, or because they have an unexpected gap in the journal in 2 months' time. From their point of view, they have nothing to lose and everything to gain.

   This does not mean that you have to agree to the idea! The editor is unlikely to lose interest in your article just because you can't deliver it a week on Friday. However, failure to meet a deadline *which you have agreed* is a much more serious issue, and the editor is likely to lose interest in you, your article and your writing career in perpetuity!

👉 **Never agree to a deadline which you think you may not be able to meet!**

Alternatively, of course, the editor may suggest a deadline 3 months away. Once again, don't agree to it unless you are sure you can deliver. If you are going to be away on holiday for 3 weeks, helping a friend with a new baby, and redecorating the spare room at weekends, 3 months may be nowhere near enough time to produce an educational article on obscure diseases of the immune system as well! On the other hand, it would not be very helpful to telephone the editor with an idea if you know you cannot deliver for 9 to 12 months. This is negotiation to meet the needs of both parties! Having agreed the deadline for submission, you can end the conversation and celebrate your success in any way you see fit.

👉 **Always make notes of what was said and agreed, either as you talk, or immediately afterwards – otherwise it is easy to forget the details of content and deadlines.**

WHAT HAPPENS NEXT?

If the editor has offered a firm commission, you will probably receive a commissioning letter from the journal, reiterating the main points of your agreement, namely the content, approach, word length and deadline. However, it is more likely that you will be left to get on with writing the article, and hear nothing more from the editor. It is not necessary to write to confirm your offer of an article. You need not write to the journal until you are submitting the finished article.

   However, you may need to call the editor again if:

● you find that you cannot write the article you promised (fire, haemorrhage and cardiac arrest are probably the only acceptable excuses for this – being 'too busy' is not. If you are that busy, you should not have offered the article in the first place)

● you find that you are unable to meet the deadline (again, only the excuses mentioned above are accepted for this)

☞ Telephone the editor *as soon as you are falling behind schedule*, **not the day before the deadline, as it is very difficult for the journal to fill the space allocated to your article at short notice.**

● you find you need to vary the content of the article (e.g. a new treatment comes out, or a new policy document is published which needs to be incorporated). In this case you need to confirm that the editor is happy for you to change the agreement you made in your previous conversation.

SUMMARY

Telephoning the editor of the journal you are targeting with your article is a very important part of the process of getting an article published. The editor has information about the planned content of the journal, and about articles that have already been commissioned, which cannot be found by reading previous issues. It also gives the editor an opportunity to mould the content and approach of your article to the journal's requirements, and so saves time which would otherwise be spent rewriting later on.

It is useful to make notes in preparation for the telephone call, and to be prepared to persuade the editor of the merits of your idea. It may be necessary to change your original idea to fit the editor's requirements, but this will greatly increase the likelihood of the article being accepted once it has been submitted to the journal.

WRITE AS YOU READ 4.1

Now prepare the notes for a conversation with the editor of your chosen journal. You have already written down the exact topic, target readership and purpose of your article, from the work you did at the end of Chapter 2. Add to this notes on:

● why you should be the person to write this article
● why this article is of interest now.

You also have the relevant editor's name and telephone number, from the research you undertook on suitable journals at the end of the last chapter. All that remains is to make that call!

Remember to have your notes to hand, and try to arrange the telephone call for a time when you have peace and privacy to talk. Write down what the editor says about content, approach, word length and deadline, so that you don't forget it when you go back to work after the call.

☞ If the first editor you approach does not like your idea, do not give up! Look at the journal assessment sheets you produced at the end of Chapter 3, and tailor your proposal to a different journal. Then ring that editor.

By the time you have finished this exercise, you should have a journal editor interested in your article. Now it is no longer just an idea in your private notepad – it is out on an editor's desk and it has a life of its own. It is the difference between planning to have a baby, and actually being pregnant. The next two chapters help you to plan for and deliver that article!

CHAPTER FIVE

PLANNING YOUR ARTICLE

The worst offence some writers commit is not structuring their article in a logical form: they just throw words down on paper. They should plan the structure before writing the article.

(*Judith Podmore, 'Nursing Management'*)

This is the final and essential preparatory step before you sit down to write your article. So far you have:

- decided exactly what to write about, for whom and why
- found a publication which reaches your target audience and takes your kind of article
- talked to the editor to make sure that they would be interested in your article.

So why not just start writing? Why spend even more time at the planning stage? As usual, the rationale is that you spend time now in order to save time later. Investing some time and thought in planning an article before writing it:

- makes the final article more coherent
- ensures that the article delivers what was agreed with the editor
- makes it easier to keep to the required word length
- allows the article to be divided into sections, which makes writing easier
- takes some of the fear out of the blank page!

As a referee for four different journals, I have reviewed many articles, both commissioned and unsolicited, before publication. I frequently see articles that appear to have been written without any attempt at planning. The content is often excellent, and there is no doubt that these articles are worth publishing for their relevance and interest to the journal's readers. However, they wander randomly through the information, backtracking and cross-referencing, and often come to an abrupt halt for no apparent reason. Sometimes there are no subheadings, just pages of dense typing, and the really interesting facts, figures and descriptions are lost in a jungle of words. There are two ways in which the reviewer can react to this type of article. One is to painstakingly identify and recommend a list of changes that would make the article acceptable for publication. These are then passed on to the author, who is invited to revise and resubmit the article. This entails a lot more work and time commitment by the author and, as often as not, this is the last time the journal or the reviewer sees that article.

☞ **If you are asked to revise your article, please do so! It means that the journal wants to publish it, and the editor and reviewer have already invested time and energy in trying to help you to be published. It is always worth the effort of making the requested revisions, because this will almost always result in publication.**

The second option for the referee is, of course, to tick the box that says 'unsuitable for publication' or, more succinctly, 'reject'. The better planned and organised an article appears, the less likely this is to happen. This chapter will look at one way of planning your article, but it is not the only way. Any method of laying out what to include, in what order and in what format, is better than none. The planning sequence described below may seem like a lot of work, but it soon becomes second nature, getting quicker and easier each time you do it.

☞ **One of the advantages of planning in this way is that you don't need to do it at your desk or in front of your computer – time in a doctor's waiting-room, on a train journey or during a period of insomnia can all be put to good use.**

FOUR STEPS IN PLANNING

The four key steps in planning your article are as follows.

Step 1: remind yourself of the aim of the article

This is important, as the purpose of the article will largely decide what information is to be included, and therefore into what sections it should be divided.

For example, if the aim of an article about diabetes is to help qualified nurses to revise their knowledge of the disease, then sections on the condition, its effect on the patient, different forms of treatment, and the nursing contribution to chronic disease management are likely to be appropriate.

However, if the aim is to give information to specialist diabetes nurses about a new form of insulin, then some of these sections might be superfluous. Instead, sections might be needed to review current forms of insulin, explain the need for a new type, and describe the differences between the new and old forms.

☞ **This part of the planning was described in Chapter 2.**

Step 2: decide on the section headings

This will help to break down the article into manageable and logical chunks for writing.

☞ **If you are writing a 2000-word article, and you have 7 sections, they only need an average of less than 300 words each. This makes the whole enterprise sound a lot less daunting.**

An article which is divided into logical sections demonstrates to the editor and the reviewer that you have taken a structured approach to your writing, which will make sub-editing and revision much easier.

Deciding on the sections also focuses your attention on the information and references you may need to have to hand before you write. For example, a description of a project might have sections headed 'Background to the project', 'Aims and objectives', 'Implementing the project', and so on, through the descriptive process. Much of this information may already exist in the form of the project plan or an existing project report. Therefore it would save much time and effort to have this written information beside you as you write the article. Alternatively, an educational article about genetically determined conditions will require some references for the statistics on prevalence that you will undoubtedly be quoting. You will need to obtain these at some stage, and it is more efficient to have them ready before you start than to leave gaps in your article which you then have to return to and fill in.

Looking at articles in the journal you are targeting will give you an idea of the number and type of sections that usually appear in their published article. Don't be afraid to mirror the article structure and section headings used. Your content will be different, so you will not be infringing any copyright, just producing a ready-to-print piece for the journal.

☞ **Don't spend a lot of time trying to find the best possible subheadings: they are likely to be changed by the journal's sub-editor anyway. Use simple, descriptive titles such as 'Background' or 'Professional issues'.**

Step 3: expand the sections

This is an opportunity to make rough notes about what each section will contain. It will help with writing the section, and also allows you to take an overview of the whole article before you start writing. If you discover at this stage that you have put too much information into the 'background' section, and left yourself little to say in the 'implementation' section, you can correct this before you have spent a lot of time writing the background.

Sketching in the content of each section will also identify the references, books or information that you need to gather before you start writing. It would be very frustrating to sit down to write a section on 'professional issues' in your article on the management of chronic asthma, only to find that you need the latest information on nurse prescribing. You then have to put off writing the section until you have found time to go to the library to look up the relevant report.

☞ **The sections don't have to be of equal length. Review the whole article plan when you have finished your notes and, if it makes a logical path towards achieving the aim of your article, then your sections are probably right.**

Step 4: take any necessary actions before you write

Now is the time to gather the books, articles, references, figures, project reports and any other information that you have identified as essential to your article.

☞ **Remember, you may also need to get permission, from a patient or your manager, to write about them or their project. It is best to do this at the earliest possible stage.**

EXAMPLES OF PLANNING

To illustrate these steps, consider three different kinds of article:

- a description of a project
- an educational article
- an opinion piece.

Example 1: the project description

Step 1: the aim of the article
'to describe how we set up an integrated care pathway for childhood asthma: aimed at nurse managers, as an example of good practice they could implement'.
Step 2: section headings
Introduction. Why childhood asthma? Integrated care pathways. The project team. Agreeing the pathway. Implementation. Making a difference. Summary.
Step 3: expanding the sections
The content of each of the sections in this article is shown in Box 5.1.
Step 4: actions arising
The actions arising from each section are shown in Box 5.2.

Box 5.1:   Integrated care pathways – expanding the sections

Section	Content
Introduction	Purpose of article
Why childhood asthma?	Prevalence figures (national); caseload profile of children with asthma; local statistics
Integrated care pathways	What they are; where they came from; references on use in other clinical areas
The project team	Principle of collaboration; how we recruited pharmacists, physiotherapists, etc.; experience of working across primary/secondary sectors
Agreeing the pathway	Process of consensus; what was agreed; summary of pathway
Implementation	Dissemination/publicity strategy; obstacles; evaluation plan
Making a difference	Findings from the evaluation; experiences of different professionals; patients' views
Summary	Difficulties; lessons learned; impact on patients

Box 5.2:   Integrated care pathways – actions

To do:

- Check with Steering Group for permission to write article
- Find national and local prevalence figures
- Literature search on integrated care pathways
- Check minutes of Steering Group meetings for details of implementation
- Ask Steering Group Chair's permission to reproduce pathway in article
- Ask audit department for help with statistics from professionals' questionnaire regarding their experiences
- Ask patients for permission to use their stories (anonymised)

Example 2: the educational article

Step 1: the aim of the article
'to describe basic urinalysis; as an educational article for nursing students, and revision for qualified nurses – part of a series of distance-learning articles'.

Box 5.3:   Urinalysis – expanding the sections

Section	Content
Aims and objectives	Purpose of article; specific learning objectives
Why test urine?	Conditions which can be diagnosed/monitored using urinalysis; advantages over blood testing
Near-patient testing	Advantages/limitations of near-patient testing; costs; equipment for urinalysis; infection control issues
Test strips and methods of use	Different test strips available; how to use them properly; interpreting results
Laboratory testing	Conditions requiring laboratory testing; different laboratory tests available and how they are carried out; cost comparison with near-patient testing
Professional issues	Patient information/advocacy/holistic care; record-keeping
Summary	Uses and advantages of urine testing
Assessment paper	2 case studies: 10 multiple-choice questions on each

Box 5.4:   Urinalysis – actions

To do:

- Check previous articles in educational series for format
- Check textbooks for conditions diagnosed/monitored with urine testing
- Send for manufacturer's information on testing strips
- Check latest infection control guidelines
- ask laboratory services directorate manager about costs of laboratory tests for urine
- Literature search on cost-comparison trials
- Check latest copy of UKCC guidance on record-keeping

Step 2: section headings
Aims and objectives of the article. Why test urine? Near-patient testing. Test strips and methods of use. Laboratory testing. Professional issues. Summary. Assessment paper.
Step 3 (expanding the sections) and Step 4 (actions arising) are shown in Boxes 5.3 and 5.4.

Example 3: the opinion piece

Step 1: the aim of the article
'to highlight the differences in nurses' knowledge about information technology, and the way it affects their practice; for general nurses, to entertain and provoke debate'
Step 2: section headings

☞ **Opinion pieces differ from most other articles in that they often do not have section headings.**

Opinion pieces are often presented as columns of text with no breaks other than paragraphs. This helps to give the impression of someone writing a letter, or talking 'off the cuff' about the topic. Such pieces are often published under headings such as 'Opinion', 'Viewpoint', 'First Person' or 'Hot Potato', implying that they are more or less spontaneous outpourings from readers or columnists. In fact, such pieces would frequently read as uncontrolled raving or mindless rambling if they were not written and edited with the same discipline as clinical articles.

☞ **This is why, despite their deceptive appearance, opinion pieces are not necessarily the easiest form of article to write.**

To stop your opinion piece falling into the 'raving or rambling' trap, you can plan it using 'invisible' section headings. These are included at the planning stage, but left out of the printed version which is submitted to the journal. To take our example, the invisible section headings could be 'Encounter with a technophobe nurse', 'Nurse "whiz kids"', 'IT developments on the wards', 'Possible Year 2050 scenario' and 'How technophobes will cope'.

Box 5.5:   Nurses and IT – expanding the sections

Section	Content
Encounter with a technophobe nurse	Story of my visit to out-patients
Nurse 'whiz kids'	Examples: Julie, Joan; language/jargon; effect on patients
IT developments on the wards	PAS, email, computerised protocols
Possible Year 2050 scenario	Virtual wards; nurse consultants on the Internet (scan in your rash and they'll diagnose it); black market in hands-on care
How technophobes will cope	Still be using list of names scribbled on paper towel?

Step 3 for this article is shown in Box 5.5.

Step 4: actions arising

There may be fewer technical actions arising from the planning of an opinion piece than for a clinical or professional article. However, facts and figures do sometimes appear, or there may be a reference to a policy document or journal article which has sparked the idea for the piece.

Sometimes other more informal actions are needed, such as talking to a few colleagues to gauge their opinion, or to elicit their experiences on the theme being discussed. Box 5.6 shows some possible actions for the example piece.

Box 5.6:   IT and nurses – actions

To do:

- Talk to Julie and Joan about examples of jargon (check spellings!)
- Look in IM&T policy document for more examples
- Check national IT strategy document for ideas about future

SUMMARY

Planning the content and layout of your article in some detail is an essential and ultimately time-saving step towards getting your article published. It is a process which can be completed in spare time, and away from the desk or computer. One approach is to look again at the aim of the article, identify the section headings and decide what to include in each section. You can then identify the books, articles or other information that you will need to gather together before starting to write. Even informal opinion pieces benefit from this planned approach.

WRITE AS YOU READ 5.1

This is the time to start the detailed planning for your article. Take the notes you made at the end of Chapter 2, and remind yourself of the aim of your article, as you summarised it.

Then draw up a box with three columns (as in Boxes 5.2, 5.4 or 5.6). Over the next few days, fill in each of the first two columns. When you are happy that these will provide a framework which will allow you to fulfil the aim of the article, complete the third column as well.

At this point, you will need to take some time to carry out the actions you have identified in the planning process. How long this takes will depend on your circumstances and on the kind of article you are writing. However, you should try to fit in these actions as soon as possible. Remember, if you have talked to an editor about your article, you may have an actual deadline to meet, or at least an editor who is vaguely looking out for a promised article. The clock has started, and you don't want to lose a great deal of time at this stage.

CHAPTER SIX

WRITING YOUR ARTICLE

Lots of editors make a decision based on the first paragraph. Sticking to a clear writing style is very impressive – plain, simple English.

(Judith Podmore, 'Nursing Management')

At last, having thought, planned, looked at journals and talked to editors, it is time to start writing! The work and time that have been put into preparing to write and planning the article should make this a much less daunting prospect than it was before. However, this is the part which no one else can do for you, so the advice and tips in this chapter are aimed at making the writing process as painless as possible.

They can be divided roughly into four categories:

- practicalities
- approach
- style
- technicalities.

☞ **Everyone has their own way of approaching writing and there is no right or wrong way. These tips concern things I have personally found helpful.**

PRACTICALITIES: GETTING STARTED

For many people, the most difficult aspect of writing an article is getting started. There are two useful steps to overcoming this problem:

- tackle the article section by section
- set yourself a deadline for each section.

☛ It is essential that your deadline for the last section is well in advance of the journal's deadline for delivery of the finished article, to allow time for revision, printing, posting, etc.

Writing one section is much more easily achieved than tackling the whole article, and the relief of completing one part gives enormous impetus to the rest! Sitting down to write 300 words on the background to your project in a spare hour is much more likely to be successful than setting aside a whole weekend and attempting to write the entire article.

☛ It is not necessary to start by writing the first section.

If the introduction is a sticking point, start with a more practical section containing facts or figures, or with the key anecdote for an opinion piece. Once this has been written, the content of the introduction will seem much more concrete, and therefore easier to write.

Another useful tip is to write to the end of a section, rather than reviewing and revising each sentence as you go. Once a section exists (on paper or on the computer), then you can go back and read it as a whole, so you can see whether the sentences, structure and train of thought make sense. The psychological boost to be gained from the fact that you have 'done' the section is very valuable! The article is no longer simply an idea, or a note on an editor's desk, but a 'work in progress'. Continuing to work on it is much easier than starting it. Some people prefer to write the whole article before reading it over. In this case, don't let the relief of having finished the article tempt you into sending it off immediately. There are nearly always some words, sentences or figures that you will find you can improve on reading through. These will jump out at you when you read the proofs before publication, but by then it will be too late to change them.

I find it much easier to read through and revise an article on paper, rather than on the computer screen. The paper version gives a much better sense of the size of each section, and how well the style is working, even though it will look different to the final layout on the journal page (see below).

PRACTICALITIES: PAPER OR COMPUTER?

One key decision about writing the article is whether to write it first on paper, before word processing, or to work directly on screen. This is an entirely personal decision, and both methods have their advantages and disadvantages (*see* Box 6.1).

☛ Choose the method which allows you to put down the most words in the shortest time. Writing quickly when preparing the first draft makes for more flowing, less stilted text.

Box 6.1:   Writing on paper versus computer

	Advantages	Disadvantages
Paper	• Can write anywhere • Cheap and easily available • No special skills required • May be quicker • Can see whole text at once • Easy to carry around	• Need to get article typed up for submission • Alterations and corrections can make text difficult to read • Difficult to move sections of text around
Computer	• Can print off article ready for submission • Easy to move text around • Can automatically correct spelling and grammatical mistakes • Alterations and corrections are invisible • May be quicker for experienced typists/word-processor users • Article can be put on disk and carried around easily	• Can only write when and where a computer is available • Need keyboard and software skills to use efficiently • Expensive if need to buy computer especially for the purpose • Work can be lost if computer crashes and no back-up is kept

---

Whichever method you use, it is helpful to:

- count words as you write (e.g. at the end of every page) – it is very frustrating to craft a well-rounded and flowing article, and then find that you have to cut or insert 1500 words afterwards (*see* Box 6.2)

Box 6.2:   Counting words

The following general guidelines may help when counting words:

- a one-page article in a nursing journal usually has around 800 words
- a half-page article usually has 400–500 words
- some journals, such as the *Health Service Journal*, have 1000 words per page, or 2000 words per two-page spread
- one page on a word processor, double-spaced with 0.5cm margins, has around 300 words.

- note in full the references you use in the text as you cite them – it is a nuisance to have to look them all up again when you have finished the article, especially if some were from library books which have since been returned.

PRACTICALITIES: PRESENTATION

As always, the journal's own Guidelines for Contributors will give detailed information about the format which best suits that particular publication. However, there are some general points which apply to the presentation of articles, whether on computer or typewriter.

- Articles should always be submitted typed or word-processed, and if you can't do this yourself, you need to find a person who can (*see* Box 6.3). Most journals ask for a copy on disk as well as a hard copy, so make sure you (or someone else) can copy the article to disk in the format required.

Box 6.3:   Getting your article typed/word-processed

To find a typist to type or word-process your manuscript:

- ask at work – some clerical staff will do typing work in the evenings for a small fee
- look on hospital or health-centre noticeboards for people advertising their word-processing services
- ask the local nursing library or University/College Department of Nursing, who may know people who type theses and assignments for students
- check small ads in the local paper, where people working from home advertise typing/word-processing services
- look in newsagents' windows, public libraries and careers or employment offices, where people who type or prepare CVs may advertise
- place your own advert in the local paper or in newsagents' windows.

Tips:

- typists usually charge either per page or per 1000 words
- if the typist is not used to preparing manuscripts for publication, it would be helpful to photocopy the Guidelines for Contributors for them
- always make a photocopy of the article before handing it over to someone else to type.

☞ **Taking a word-processing course yourself would be an enormously valuable investment!**

Box 6.4:   Formatting articles on computer

The Guidelines for Contributors will give detailed guidance, but the following general points can be applied:

- leave wide margins on both sides of the page for the editor's and sub-editor's comments and alterations
- use double-spacing (unless specifically instructed otherwise in the Guidelines)
- include a separate title page with author's details, and don't repeat your name on the other pages
- number all of the pages
- justify to the left, but leave the right margin unjustified
- use devices such as bold type, italics and underlining sparingly and consistently
- use only one or two different sizes or styles of heading
- use a standard font and font size (e.g. Times New Roman, 12 point)
- use the tabulation key, not the space bar, to indent
- put only one space after punctuation marks (including full stops)
- use only one return between paragraphs and between sections.

- When using a computer (or instructing someone word-processing on your behalf), use minimum formatting (*see* Box 6.4). Remember that the layout of the article on the journal page will be quite different to your original text, and will be made to conform to the 'house style' of the journal. Any fancy formatting you put in will have to be taken out again at the sub-editing stage!
- Put the list of references, and each box, figure or diagram, on a separate page at the end of the article – don't insert them into the text. Again, they will all be redrawn or redrafted in house to conform to the journal's style, and they may need to be separated and sent off to different people for this to be done.

☞ **Make sure that each figure is clearly numbered and titled, so that it can be linked up again with the correct part of the correct article (yours!) after this process.**

Box 6.5:   What to put on the title page

- Article title
- Names of all authors
- Professional and academic qualifications (*not* English National Board courses, dates of qualifications, PIN numbers)
- Positions and places of work of all authors
- Address, telephone and fax numbers of the leading author
- email address of the leading author, if applicable
- Number of words in the manuscript

- Attach a title page to your manuscript, giving your name, address and other relevant details (*see* Box 6.5).
- Don't put your name on each page, as papers are sent anonymously to referees, and someone will have to remove your name from each page before doing this! Identify the article by its title in a 'footer' at the bottom of the page instead.
- Number the pages of the article, to help with reassembly after they have been photocopied for the referees.

APPROACH

The most important guide to the approach to any article is the Guidelines for Contributors for the journal. This will set out any required section headings, particularly for articles about research studies or project reports, and will also often give very clear hints about the line to take in presenting your information.

For example, the 'Information for Authors' from *Primary Health Care Research and Development* states that 'all papers should make clear the potential application of their content to practice, and where possible points should be summarised in text boxes'.

The *Health Service Journal*, on its page entitled 'How to submit articles', states that 'we are always ready to consider topical material and publicise examples of good practice which have been in operation for at least six months and demonstrated quantifiable benefits to patients. We favour detailed accounts of practical local approaches to common management issues which will have lessons for managers elsewhere. Articles should be comprehensible to readers without a specialist knowledge'.

This particular journal goes on to specify the number of words, diagrams and references which can be included in the article, the method of referencing, the content of research reports and case studies, and detailed instructions for presentation. With the approach so clearly defined, the author is left with nothing to do but fill in the words!

An additional source of guidance on the approach to take to your article consists of the recently published articles in the same journal. Looking specifically at similar articles to your own, you may notice that, for example:

- they use lots of bullet points, or
- clinical articles often start with the story of a particular patient, or
- they place most emphasis on the disease/treatment/technical aspects rather than patient experience, or
- opinion pieces usually state both sides of an argument, or
- authors use the first person ('I/we decided' rather than 'it was decided'), or
- they use lots of diagrams and figures.

Any of these characteristics (and many others) can be a useful pointer to the approach you should use. After all, you are looking at articles which were published, so they obviously represent exactly the type of approach which the journal favours.

☞ **Don't be afraid to mimic a successful approach – there is no copyright on the approach, only on the words!**

The exception to this rule is humorous articles, when the approach is not only very individual to the writer, but is part of the humour, too. It would be difficult to copy, and would also be highly likely to be rejected by the editor as a pale imitation of the original writer.

Almost all articles in all publications are divided into sections by subheadings. Use them frequently to break up the text, including that in the main sections of the article. A number of short sections are easier to read and digest than a few long ones. For research reports, there are some commonly used standard subheadings (*see* Box 6.6). Otherwise it is left to the author to break up the text appropriately.

☞ **Keep subheadings simple, as they are quite likely to be changed at the sub-editing stage.**

Box 6.6:   Usual subheadings for research papers

Introduction
(Aim)
Methods
Results
Discussion
Conclusion
(Acknowledgements)
References

Brief research reports:

Aim
Methods
Findings
References (usually limited to 3–4)

Graphs, figures, tables, drawings and photographs are also useful for breaking up the text. The Guidelines for Contributors may limit the number you can use, or a scan of similar published articles in the same journal may show that they like to use many of these devices in preference to long descriptions in the text. They can also be useful for presenting a lot of information without using up too much of the word allocation, if an article is threatening to become too long.

☞ **It is important not to repeat information that is contained in tables or graphs in the text. Simply refer to the table.**

STYLE

Writing style is a very personal attribute, and some writers are easily identifiable by their style, even if they are writing anonymously. For opinion pieces or humorous articles, style is everything, and editors will accept some very idiosyncratic approaches. However, when you are first submitting clinical or educational articles to journals, it is probably best to maintain a more conventional style.

The following suggestions are aimed at helping to reinforce a basic, conventional writing style for purely practical purposes, rather than stifling individuality. Conventional wisdom includes the following tips.

Keep sentences short

This is a particularly difficult rule for me to follow: I have a definite preference for long sentences, which seem to me to be essential to convey the ideas I want to include; they contain frequent sub-clauses, elaborating on the general theme, and I have to use almost every punctuation device in the language to render them readable at all! (See what I mean?) However, sub-editors will cut down long sentences into short ones, if you don't, and the result can seem rather stilted. It is better to provide the short sentences yourself, and to ensure that the passage reads smoothly.

Avoid excessive formality

The articles I am sent to review sometimes contain incredibly complex language and sentence structure. It is as if the author feels that 'ordinary' language is not good enough for an article for publication, and he or she therefore adopts a strange formal style instead. Reading published articles in the journal you are targeting will give a good idea of the degree of formality required in the writing (and it is usually minimal).

Avoid excessive informality

There is always an opposite end to the spectrum, and in this case it is the article written like a conversation over a garden fence. Unless you are deliberately satirising that approach to the topic in a humorous piece, such informality is not usually appropriate. Again, previously published articles are a good guide to the journal's style. As a general example:

- Too formal: 'One has frequently postulated the merits of universal prescribing within the nursing profession'

- Too informal: 'How many times have we asked ourselves "Why, oh why, can't all nurses be allowed to prescribe?"'
- Try instead: 'There has been a lot of debate about nurse prescribing'.

☞ **A commonly quoted rule of thumb is 'Write as you talk'. Take this with a pinch of salt if your speaking style has ever been described as 'colourful'!**

Don't describe in words what could be better shown in figures

Delivering the results of a survey, or figures on the uptake of a service, in long paragraphs of text makes the article unnecessarily difficult for the reader to follow. As well as being unattractive on the page (and so liable to being revised by the editor on aesthetic grounds), it is difficult to grasp the significance of numerical data when it is described in words. Graphs and pie charts display information much more effectively, and make a greater impact on the reader.

☞ **Don't repeat in the text any information that is contained in figures or charts. Just refer to it by saying, for example, 'The age and sex breakdown of participants is shown in Figure 1'.**

Don't worry if you have problems with pie charts and graphs on the computer. You can always hand-draw them, as they will have to be redrawn in house anyway.

TECHNICALITIES

Spelling

Some journals specify whether they want American English or British English spellings. This particularly affects words such as 'specialisation' (or 'specialization') and 'theatre' (or 'theater'). However, if there is no guidance, do not worry too much about it. The journal will make any necessary alterations. For general spelling, use the computer spell-check facility, but also check the text visually. The computer check will pass words which may be wrongly spelt in the context, but do appear in the dictionary. This can lead to alarming statements such as 'beast-feeding provides the baby with additional antibodies' and 'some asthma drugs slow down the heart rat'. While a few of these may brighten an editor's day, too many suggest a careless approach to the article as a whole.

Drug names

Some publications provide explicit guidance on the use of drug names. This usually involves giving the generic name (rather than the brand name) of the product or, where brand names have to be used, giving all of the possible alternatives, in order to avoid endorsing one particular product. Needless to say, it is essential to be accurate in giving dosages, and in particular to differentiate between micrograms and milligrams, by using the full word rather than abbreviations.

Numbers

Most Guidelines for Contributors ask that numbers one to ten are written as words, while numbers from 11 upward are expressed as figures. An exception usually occurs when the figures would appear at the beginning of a sentence: '24 questionnaires were returned' does not look as neat as 'Twenty-four questionnaires. . .'.

Some journals may also require percentages to be written as '20 per cent' rather than '20%'. Remember, though, that most numerical data has more impact when presented as charts or tables, rather than as text.

Punctuation

This causes many people unnecessary concern. The only reason for worrying about 'getting it right' is to appear reasonably literate and educated, in order to establish some credibility with the editor. However, the sub-editor will change and correct as necessary so, if you are concerned, revise the basics (see Appendix B) and then get on with the important part – writing the article.

Paragraphing

This is definitely at the mercy of both the sub-editor and the amount of space in the column. Put in plenty of paragraphs at the writing stage, as it makes the article look more professional and attractive on the page. However, you must be prepared for it to look very different in the printed version. If you are particularly concerned to keep some of your paragraph breaks, make the contents different sections, separated by a new subheading – this may have some protective effect!

References

These probably cause more anxiety to the writer, and more irritation to the reviewer and editor, than all of the other technical issues together. It seems obvious to state that references should be:

- in the style (usually Vancouver or Harvard) specified by the journal
- listed at the end of the article on a separate page
- limited to the number of references allowed by the journal
- complete, with every citation in the text matched with a full reference in the list at the end of the article

- accurate with regard to names, dates and publication details
- primary rather than secondary sources.

However, the majority of articles which I review for journals do not meet one or other (or sometimes any) of these criteria. I have seen an article with more than 60 references in the text (far too many for the journal to print), and 16 of these missing from the reference list at the end. Another article used almost entirely secondary references, several of them from articles I had written, to substantiate some very contentious claims. Where I had quoted the original source for the statements, this author's referencing implied that it was I who had made the claims! That manuscript went back to the journal with some very indignant comments, and a firm recommendation for revisions prior to publication.

Some other common problems with referencing are shown in Box 6.7. (For a reminder about the correct methods of referencing, *see* Appendix C.)

Box 6.7:   Common errors in referencing

Missing information
For example, the place of publication of a book (can be found on the title page); volume and issue numbers for journals (e.g. reference cites '*Nursing Standard*, March 3 1999' instead of the correct '*Nursing Standard*, vol 13, no. 24') (this information appears at the foot of each page of the journal)

Secondary, rather than primary, sources cited
For example, reference is 'Jones, 1998' saying that x per cent of the population of England is of Asian ethnic origin, when in fact Jones cites the original census data (the primary source). The author should cite the census, not Jones

Out-of-date sources cited
For example, using census data from the 1980 census, when the 1990 data is available (unless the writer is specifically referring to the situation as it was in 1980). Older references may be appropriate if they are the seminal works on a topic (e.g. Schon, 1983, on reflective practice in nursing) or if they are likely to be unchanged (e.g. works on anatomy and physiology, provided that recent technological developments or scientific experiments have not revealed new facts or understanding which ought to be included). Current references (less than 3 years old) are usually essential in articles discussing professional developments, although older references may be appropriate when describing the background to those developments

---

For foolproof referencing:
- write out the references in full, in the journal's style, when you first come across them during your research or reading

- keep this list around when you are writing, and number the references on the list as you cite them in the text
- write out the article's reference list when you have finished the body of the text, by listing the numbered references, in either numerical or alphabetical order, depending which system the journal requires
- avoid using the phrase 'cited in', quoting a reference quoted in another publication. Give the details of the original publication.

Language

Many journals accept and indeed encourage international contributions. Experience from other countries and healthcare systems is often very valuable to the development of nursing. However, if English is not your first language, some journals' Guidelines for Contributors ask authors to have the manuscript read by a native English speaker prior to submission.

Gender-neutral language

This has become an issue for nursing journals as for every other form of publication, and editors expect authors to use appropriate terms in their articles.

The clumsy forms of 'she/he' and '(s)he' have fallen from favour, and other alternatives are preferred. Try, for example:

- changing from the singular to the plural – so 'the editor will tell you what he is looking for' becomes 'editors will tell you what they are looking for'
- changing key nouns – so 'Chairman' becomes 'Chair'
- avoiding unnecessary gender labelling, such as 'male nurse'.

There is no need to use the convoluted, sometimes ludicrous circumlocutions favoured by comedians who are making fun of political correctness. Simple devices such as those mentioned above soon become second nature, and will add to the professionalism of your writing.

Patients' names

Patient or client names should be changed to protect their confidentiality, and it is worth stating that this has been done at the end of the article. If the editor considers that this policy is sufficiently well known, the statement can always be edited out before publication.

Permissions

It is usual to obtain a patient's permission before writing about their case in an article, even if their name is to be changed. Managers may require a note of the conversation with the patient to be recorded.

It is essential to obtain permission if you want to reproduce a diagram, figure or drawing from another publication in your article. You will need to write to the editor (of a journal) or the publishers (of a book) for permission, stating exactly which item you want to use, for what purpose, and where you hope to be published. You should also ask what form of acknowledgement the editor or publisher requires in the new publication. When you receive a reply giving permission, copy this letter and send it to the editor with your article.

✍ **This is equivalent to putting in a reference when you quote text from someone else's work. Not to do so implies to the reader that you produced the diagram or figure yourself, and is a form of plagiarism.**

STARTING TO WRITE: APPLYING THE GUIDANCE

EXAMPLE 1

Imagine that the following paragraph is from the first draft of an article describing a project working with homeless people. It is aimed at community nurses, as an example of good practice, and targeted at *Primary Health Care*, the community nursing journal produced by the Nursing Standard's publishing company.

Draft 1

This might read:

> *Setting up the project*
> *As the project involved district nurses, practice nurses and health visitors travelling around the city providing care, advice and support to people living on the streets, it was important that all the agencies who needed to be involved were represented on the steering group, based in the Trust, which oversaw the implementation of the project. The aims of the project were to provide any necessary clinical care to people living on the street, to provide advice about welfare and other benefits available to the clients, to liaise with other local care givers and health professionals (such as GPs and voluntary services) as necessary, and to integrate clients into mainstream primary care services whenever possible. The members of the Steering Group therefore consisted of a local GP, a representative of social services, a representative from the local drugs and alcohol service, a Trust nurse manager, a public health specialist and a housing officer from the local authority. The Steering Group had to consider issues such as the safety of the nurses, the practical issues of running the vehicle, long-term funding for the project after the 'pump-priming' funding finished and the evaluation of the project.*

The content of this paragraph is fine, but the approach, style and technicalities need some attention. Each sentence consists of a list, and the sentences tend to be rather long. There is nothing to break up the long run of plain text, and no variation in the appearance of the paragraph on the page. If the paragraph was revised following some of the suggestions in this chapter, it might read as follows.

Draft 2

Setting up the project

The aims of the project were:

- *to provide any necessary clinical care to people living on the street*
- *to provide advice about welfare and other benefits available to the clients*
- *to liaise with other local caregivers and health professionals (such as GPs and voluntary services) as necessary*
- *to integrate clients into mainstream primary care services whenever possible.*

The project involved district nurses, practice nurses and health visitors travelling around the city providing care, advice and support to people living on the streets. It was important, therefore, that all the agencies who needed to be involved were represented on the Trust-based steering group which oversaw the implementation of the project. The members of the Steering Group are shown in Figure 1. [A simple box, with the membership listed by profession]

The Steering Group had to consider issues such as:

- *the safety of the nurses*
- *the practical issues of running the vehicle*
- *long-term funding for the project after the 'pump-priming' funding finished*
- *the evaluation of the project.*

In this revised version, the same information is conveyed in a more attractive format. Bullet-point lists of the aims of the project, and of the issues considered by the steering group, break up the text. The information is also easier to assimilate when it is presented as a list. The list of steering group members has been removed from the text, to avoid having three bullet-point lists very close together, and to provide visual variety on the page.

EXAMPLE 2

Imagine that the following paragraph is from an article describing an audit of discharge planning procedures. It is aimed at nurses, managers and audit co-ordinators working in acute and long-stay units, and targeted at an audit journal.

Draft 1

This might read:

> *Results*
>
> *At the time of the first audit, only 17 (36 per cent) general surgical in-patients had a written discharge plan, compared to 20 (47 per cent) gynaecological patients and 18 (50 per cent) patients on the long-stay elderly care unit. The Trust guidelines state that all patients should have a written discharge plan in their hospital records: the standard against which the records were compared was therefore 100%. At re-audit, 12 months later, 19 (40 per cent) surgical patients, 18 (46 per cent) gynaecological patients and 27 (75%) elderly care patients had written discharge plans. Fifteen patient records could not be traced during the first audit, and 11 records could not be traced at re-audit. In the staff survey carried out at the same time as the two audits, seven ward managers, 11 F-grade staff nurses, nine E-grade staff nurses and eight D-grade staff nurses were asked about their awareness of, and attitude to, the Trust guidelines on discharge planning. While 95% of the staff nurses claimed to have seen the guidelines 'recently' or 'very recently', only three of the seven ward managers had done so.*

Again, the information contained in this paragraph is exactly what the reader wants to know. However, there is a lot of detailed information contained in rather dense text with long sentences, and figures and percentages are scattered throughout. Words and figures are used inconsistently, and percentages are variously described using 'per cent' and '%'. It would be very difficult for the reader to grasp the significance of the results, or even to remember what had been measured. This paragraph could be revised as follows.

Draft 2

> *Results*
>
> *The Trust guidelines state that all patients (100 per cent) should have a written discharge plan in their hospital records. This was the standard against which the records were compared. Results for the general surgical, gynaecological and long-stay elderly care units are shown in Figure 1 [a single bar chart displaying the three units' results, at audit and re-audit, against a 100 per cent standard. A note at the bottom of the chart states the number of missing records at each audit]. The elderly care unit achieved the highest percentage of patients with care plans in their records at both the original audit and the re-audit. It was also the only unit to show significant improvement over the 12 months of the audit period.*
>
> *A survey of 35 members of staff was carried out at the same time as the two audits. The staff groups involved in the survey are shown in Figure 2 [pie chart showing each staff group as a percentage of the whole survey population]. Staff*

awareness of the discharge planning guidelines varied considerably between grades (see Figure 3) [bar chart(s) showing different groups' responses to the awareness questions], with D- and E-grade staff nurses more likely to have seen the Trust guidelines 'recently' than higher-grade staff.

In this revised version, most of the numbers and percentages have been replaced by bar and pie charts, which can contain all of the information (numbers, percentages, units, original audit figures, re-audit figures etc.) in one visual display. This allows space in the text to draw attention to the most interesting or significant results.

COLLABORATING

It is very much a matter of personal opinion whether it is easier to produce an article on your own, or by collaborating with one or more other people. My own preference is to write alone, because:

- the time-scale is under my control – I can accept long or short deadlines as it suits me, and work around my other commitments
- I don't have to compromise on content, style or approach
- articles flow easily and logically, without artificial or abrupt changes in style.

However, there are advantages to collaborating:

- the discipline helps to ensure that deadlines are met
- large pieces of work become much more manageable when you are only responsible for some of the writing
- different perspectives and expertise add additional authority and interest to the article.

There are different ways of collaborating on an article (*see* Box 6.8), which will be appropriate in different situations. In cases where a large number of people have been involved in a project, for example, it may be sensible for one person to draft the article so that the others can then comment and make suggestions for redrafting.

For an educational article about a particular condition, it might make more sense for one person to write the section on the condition, while another describes the nursing input to treatment and management.

Whichever method of collaboration you choose, it is important to allow enough time for all parties to read and approve the final draft.

☛ **At a conservative estimate, collaboration probably takes at least twice as long as writing an article alone!**

Box 6.8: Different ways of collaborating on articles

Author plus reviewers

One person drafts the article, and the other(s) then read through the draft and suggest corrections, additions or changes. The original writer amends the draft, and all of them review and revise later drafts until they agree that they are satisfied with the article.

Co-authors

Two or more people plan the article and then divide the content between them. Each author writes some sections of the article, which are then reviewed by the other(s). In addition to suggesting amendments, all of the authors need to ensure that the style is consistent throughout the article.

Author plus contributor

One person writes the text of the article. They then invite someone else to contribute a short piece (perhaps 100–200 words) to be added as a self-contained box or panel (e.g. a case study, an example of good practice, a personal experience, a different perspective, or a different professional's view).

Ghost writer

One person describes what they want to say, makes notes and discusses it with the ghost writer. The latter produces a draft of the article, which they amend following comments and corrections from the first person. The article is offered for publication in the name of the first individual.

When an article is multi-authored, the journal will usually ask you to identify a 'lead author' to whom their correspondence should be addressed. It is worth sorting this out early in the writing process, as you may reach a point where someone has to make the final decisions on issues such as when the article is ready for submission.

SUMMARY

Writing an article is a much less daunting task if some research and planning have been undertaken first. The Guidelines for Contributors produced by the targeted journal provide the best source of guidance on approach and style, as well as detailed instructions on formatting, spelling and referencing. Previously published articles in the journal also provide ideas on style, and can be used as informal templates for new articles (*see* Appendix D). It is usually helpful to write a first draft fairly quickly so that the words and ideas flow smoothly and logically. This can then be revised as necessary to ensure that it is readable, fully referenced and attractively laid out. If an article is to be written in collaboration with others, it is likely to take considerably longer than a single-author piece. An appropriate method of working has to be identified which will ensure that the journal's deadlines are met.

WRITE AS YOU READ 6.1

Now it is time to write that article! Have close at hand:

- the journal's Guidelines for Contributors
- the notes of your conversation with the editor about content, length, etc.
- a recent copy of the journal featuring a similar article to your own
- the plan you prepared at the end of Chapter 5.

Choose the section which you think will be easiest to write, and set aside a short period of time (1–2 hours) to write it.

☛ **Remember, the introduction can be much more difficult to write than a section with more 'solid' content.**

Whether you are writing on paper or on computer, try to write the section fairly quickly. Avoid the temptation to revise and correct as you go, as this will interrupt the flow of words. Then repeat the process with the other sections. For some articles, it helps to take the main sections in order, even if you add the introduction later, while others will have several discrete sections which can be written in any order. Don't forget to count the words in each section as you write them.

☛ **When you are writing, don't let a missing reference or statistic, or the need for a chart or graph, halt the flow. Miss it out for now, and fill it in later.**

Once you have written all the sections, print them out (if using a computer) and then read the article through as a whole. Check that it is logical in layout, clear in meaning and easy to read on the page. Compare it with some of the articles in the journal to check that it is not totally different in style and approach.

Once you have made any necessary revisions to the body of the text, you can add the reference list and any figures (charts, graphs, boxes, lists, etc.) to which you referred in the text. Remember that these will need to be printed/typed on a separate page each and placed at the end of the article.

Finally, count the words for the last time, check the spelling, and double-check the reference list and figures.

At this point some people would advocate putting the article away for a couple of weeks and then rereading it. However, I suspect that no one would ever get round to sending their article to a journal if they followed this advice too closely. Every time you look at your manuscript you will see something else that you could alter. If you have read through and revised the article, and you are happy that it does what you intended it to do, then you might as well send it off.

Another common suggestion is to ask a colleague to read through the article and make suggestions for changes or improvements. The risks of this strategy are that they will either be too kind to suggest anything, in which case you have wasted time to no purpose, or they will have ideas for improvement which you then have to accept (involving altering the manuscript) or reject (involving altering your relationship with your colleague, perhaps forever). The choice is yours.

☛ **You may need to share the manuscript with colleagues if you are writing about a joint project, or if you need your manager's permission to submit the article.**

CHAPTER SEVEN

MORE THINGS TO DO BEFORE PUBLICATION

It's really good if the author can supply the article on disk. And good-quality photos are very useful – it's very difficult to find the right pictures to illustrate an article from a picture library.

(Clare Parker, 'Practice Nurse')

Don't ring after two days and ask what's happening. Check the authors' guidelines to see how long the process takes. Add on a week, then ring.

(Daniel Allen, 'Mental Health Nursing')

Unfortunately for the busy writer, your work does not finish with the completion of your article. There are still a lot of steps between submission of the finished article and publication (*see* Figure 7.1), and the writer has an essential contribution to make to several of them.

PREPARING THE ARTICLE FOR DISPATCH

The first step following the final revisions and completion of the article is of course to prepare it for dispatch to the journal. Once again, the journal's Guidelines for Contributors are essential for guidance. Most publications ask for articles to be submitted on paper and on disk, but the number of hard (paper) copies that they require can vary from one to three or four.

THE DISK COPY

☞ It is essential that the version of the article on the disk matches the version on the paper printout exactly. Ensure that late revisions appear on both versions.

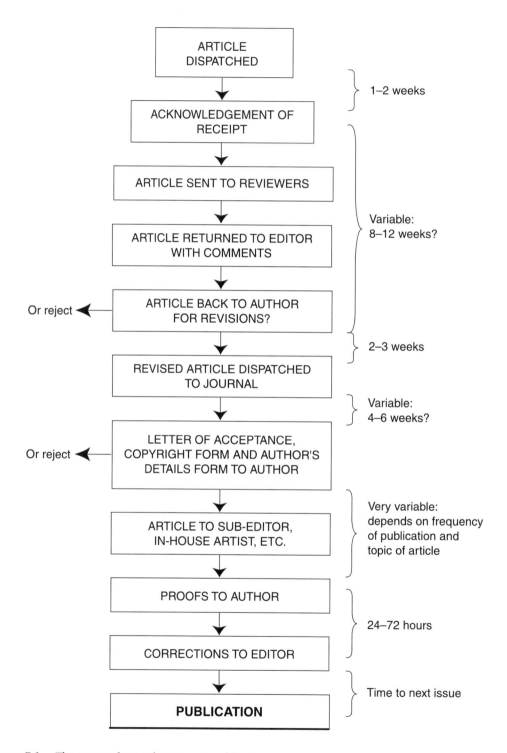

Figure 7.1:   The process from submission to publication.

When preparing the disk for dispatch, ensure that it is clearly and indelibly labelled with:

- your name and address
- the title of the article
- the word-processing package and version used to produce the document.

Sometimes the Guidelines for Contributors ask for the document to be saved in ASCII or text form. This is a generic form which will enable the article to be read by any word-processing package, as the one used by the journal may well be different to that used by the writer. Instructions for saving the document in this way can usually be found in the 'Help' index of your word-processing package.

THE HARD COPY

☞ **Use good-quality paper (80 grams or higher) for printing out your article, as lighter paper becomes dog-eared very easily as it is being handled in the journal's office.**

Use a paper clip rather than a staple to fasten the pages together, as they may have to be photocopied to be sent out to reviewers. Make sure that the pages are numbered, though, so that the article can be easily reassembled if the clip should part company with the paper at some point!

OTHER THINGS TO INCLUDE

If you have any good-quality, colour photographs which could accompany your article, these will be gratefully received by the editor. In the absence of photographs supplied by the author, the editor will have to rely on picture libraries (these pictures may be out of date, inappropriate or simply unattractive, and they cause many letters of complaint from readers, and much disgruntlement among members of editorial boards).

If in your article you have used a table or figure which has been taken from another book or article, you will have to obtain permission to reproduce it by writing to the original publishers. A copy of their letter to you, granting the permission, should be sent to the journal with your article.

DISPATCHING THE ARTICLE

The usual method of dispatch is the traditional one – the postal system. If you are writing a short opinion piece (200–300 words) to a very tight deadline (days rather than weeks), the editor may ask you to fax it to the journal, but this is the exception rather than the rule. In general, unless asked to do so, you should not fax your article to the journal. Moreover, while email is useful for contacting the editor with queries or messages, it is not generally used to send in articles for publication.

In preparation for posting, it is worth obtaining some reasonably strong envelopes in A4 size for articles of several thousand words, or A5 size for brief pieces. Cheaper, lighter envelopes can be damaged on the way to the journal editor's office, and slightly damp or crumpled manuscripts do not make the best impression on the editor.

☞ **Remember, you can only submit your article to one journal at a time.**

In the letter to the editor that accompanies the article, there is the opportunity to repeat the selling points you made in your telephone conversation weeks or months previously. The editor may well have forgotten why they expressed an interest in your piece on continence problems in postnatal women or, indeed, who you are and why you are writing to them. You can use the letter to remind the editor that National Continence Day is coming up in 6 months' time and, as a practice nurse, you are often consulted by women about stress incontinence after childbirth. You can also remind the editor that you discussed the article with them on the telephone, and that you have taken into account the suggestions (about word length, content or approach) that they made. This is where your notes on the original conversation are very useful.

Just like the presentation of the article, the letter to the editor needs to give a good, professional impression of you as a writer. It is helpful to get it typed or word-processed, together with your article.

With the article on disk and printed out on paper, and the letter to accompany it, the final pre-dispatch check-list looks like this.

- Is the article in the correct format for the journal?
- Are the correct number of paper copies enclosed?
- Is a fully labelled disk enclosed, containing an identical copy of the article?
- Is a professional and persuasive letter to the editor enclosed?
- Are all other necessary items included with the article (e.g. photos, permissions)?
- Has a good-quality envelope been used?
- Is the full and correct address of the journal, together with the name and designation of the editor, marked clearly on the envelope?
- Is there sufficient postage on the envelope (anything more than two sheets of paper and a disk will cost more than the standard first-class letter postage)?

☞ **Before posting, check that you have a complete copy of the article for yourself, preferably on the computer as well as on paper. Articles can and do get lost in the post!**

It is not necessary to send articles by recorded delivery. They are no more likely to arrive in this way, although it does allow you to phone and check that the letter has arrived at its destination.

ACKNOWLEDGEMENT

Most journals acknowledge the arrival of a manuscript by sending out a postcard or letter. This often arrives within a couple of days, or at most a week or two, after dispatch of the article. Its purpose is simply to acknowledge receipt, and it does not imply anything more than this. If you don't receive such an acknowledgement, and you would like to be reassured that your article has arrived, you could telephone the editor to check.

☞ **Don't ask the editor for even a preliminary opinion at this early stage: confine yourself to checking that the article has arrived and then say goodbye!**

REVIEWING/REFEREEING OF ARTICLES

Although, as the writer, you are not directly involved in this step towards publication, it is useful to know what happens to your article. Journals which are 'peer-reviewed' have a panel of reviewers or referees (the words are frequently used interchangeably) to whom articles are sent by the editor for review. Reviewers may be experts in the clinical field covered by the journal, or they may have qualifications or experience relevant to the types of article that the journal wishes to publish (e.g. an education-alist for a journal that publishes distance-learning articles).

☞ **The names of the review panel are sometimes published on the same page as the list of editors and staff of the journal.**

Each article is usually sent to one or two referees for an opinion. Articles on very specialised topics may also be sent to suitably qualified or experienced people who are not on the formal panel of referees, for an additional expert opinion. Much of the delay between an article arriving on the editor's desk and a decision being conveyed to the author is caused by the need to send the article out to one or more expert reviewers.

The review panel has a particularly important role to play when the editor and staff of a journal are journalists rather than nurses (or other health professionals). The reviewers can advise on issues of professional and clinical importance which might otherwise be missed or misinterpreted.

The reviewers' role in relation to the article is to assess the relevance, quality and accuracy of the content.

- *Relevance* relates to whether the article will be of interest to the publication's readers, and whether the topic is sufficiently new, interesting or important to be featured in the journal.
- *Quality* includes the quality of information in the article – whether it is up to date, comprehensive and at the right level for the readership – as well as the way in which it is presented.
- *Accuracy* relates to the technical information contained in the article, the statements and claims made by the author, and the accuracy of the referencing.

☛ **The preparation and planning that preceded the writing of the article should ensure safe passage through the review stage.**

Reviewers are sometimes paid a small sum for giving an opinion on an article, but many are not. They are busy professionals who fit in reviewing articles alongside many other commitments. A well-written and well-presented article will make a good impression on the busy reviewer as well as on the editor. Articles are usually reviewed 'blind' – that is, the reviewer is not given the author's name, nor is the author told who has reviewed their article. The reviewer's comments may be photocopied and sent to the author, or summarised in a letter or telephone call from the editor.

REVISIONS

It is very common for articles to be returned to the editor from the reviewers with requests for some revision by the author. The revisions requested may be:

- a change in emphasis or approach
- the inclusion of additional material or sections
- changes to technical aspects, such as completing references, checking facts or correcting misleading statements.

There are three easy rules for approaching revisions:

- make them!
- do this quickly and professionally
- if you are not happy with the suggested revisions, talk to the editor and then do whatever you have agreed.

It is very frustrating for editors and reviewers alike when articles sent back to authors for revision disappear, never to be seen again. It is still worse, as described in an earlier chapter, if they reappear unchanged at a different journal, where the reviewer makes exactly the same requests for revision!

☞ **If an editor or reviewer asks for revisions, they are seriously interested in publishing your article. Capitalise on this interest, and you will have a published article!**

It is entirely understandable that, after spending precious time and effort writing the article, you don't want to have to think about it again. However, the work involved in revision is minimal compared to starting again with a new article. Editors, and particularly sub-editors, will put a lot of effort of their own into shaping your article so that it is suitable for publication – you only need to give them the basic material. Thus it is always worth supplying that extra section, or checking the reference, and resubmitting the article as quickly as possible.

If the requested revision is a change in emphasis or approach, don't despair – this does not mean that you have to do a complete rewrite. Suppose you have written a 2000-word article on clinical governance, aimed at community nurses, for a community nursing journal. The reviewer comments that the content is excellent but very general, and that it needs to be more focused on community nursing.

Rather than rewriting the whole article, you could:

- put some examples relevant to community nurses in boxes, to be printed alongside the text
- replace the word 'nurse' with 'community nurse' in some or all of the article
- change the references so that readers are directed to other articles concerning community nurses' quality and audit work, rather than more general sources.

None of these approaches would take very long or mean discarding anything you had already written. However, you would have acceded to the reviewer's requests and you would be almost certain of publication.

What happens if you disagree strongly with the reviewer's assessment of your article? I have been in this position, when a reviewer sent pages of suggested alterations to an educational article I had written. Some of the suggestions were helpful, and I made the necessary changes quite happily. Other suggestions seemed to me to miss the point of the article entirely, and one or two seemed downright perverse! I discussed the reviewer's comments with the editor, and we agreed which would be implemented and which could be set aside.

☞ **It is always worth discussing any concerns about reviewers' comments with the editor, rather than simply giving up on the article. Reviewers are not infallible.**

ACCEPTANCE

At some point in the process you will receive an acceptance letter from an editor. If you have talked to the editor before writing the article, studied the target journal carefully, tailored your article to the publication and responded positively to the reviewer's comments, your article will probably be accepted by the first journal to which you sent it.

If it should be rejected, perhaps because of some major policy change which has altered the journal's priorities, you will have selected a different journal, revised your article appropriately and resubmitted it. Therefore, sooner or later, you will receive the acceptance letter.

There are likely to be two forms to complete, which either come with the acceptance letter or are sent on later:

- a copyright form
- an author's details form.

The copyright form will ask you to sign over the copyright of your article to the journal. As the journals will only publish articles submitted exclusively to them, and they expect to have the copyright, there is no point in arguing with this. Read the form so that you understand exactly which rights you are giving to the journal, and then sign and return it.

Signing over copyright of the article to the journal does not mean that you lose all contact with your article. Journal publishers are happy to give permission for your article to be reproduced in other places – such as books – by you or other people, provided that permission is sought first and they are acknowledged as the copyright holder. I have had some journal articles which originally appeared in *Nursing Standard* reprinted in the *Guardian* newspaper, and others included in a compilation of humour in nursing, published in the USA. In each case, the editors approached the editor of *Nursing Standard*, rather than me, to ask for permission to reprint the articles.

I have also asked permission from the journal *Practice Nurse* to reuse a diagram from one of my articles in a book chapter I have contributed to a multi-authored book. The editor was happy to give me the necessary permission, and the diagram will appear with an acknowledgement to its first published source.

☞ **Remember that the copyright of the article belongs to the journal, once you have signed the copyright form. If you are approached for permission to reprint some or all of the article, you must direct the enquirer to the journal.**

The author's details form has to be completed because the journal production staff need to know your full name, designation, place of work and relevant academic and professional qualifications, in order to print these at the beginning or end of your article.

☞ **You do not need to give dates or PINs for any of your qualifications, just the letters that you want to appear after your name.**

The form will usually also ask for your daytime telephone and fax numbers, and your email address if you have one, so that the editor can communicate with you quickly during the preparation stage of your article. Some journals also ask if there is any period when you are going to be unavailable (e.g. on holiday) because of the urgency attached to proof-reading (see below).

PROOF-READING

The proofs of your article are in effect a preview of the article as it will be printed. There are two types of proofs:

- galley proofs, which are simply columns of print
- page proofs, which show the layout of the article as it will appear on the page, usually complete with tables and diagrams.

Most journals will send a copy of the page proofs of an article to the author for checking before publication. The exceptions are opinion pieces, humorous pieces and regular columns, which are usually printed without checking by the author.

☞ **The purpose of proof-reading is to correct technical errors such as misspellings, incorrect drug dosages, etc. It is not an opportunity to add to or alter the text.**

Proofs are sent to the author, often by fax, very shortly before the journal goes to press. The deadline for corrections to be notified to the editor or sub-editor is usually very short (24–48 hours is common).

☞ **It is essential that you telephone the named person before this deadline expires. Otherwise, it will be too late, and you will have to deal with the consequences if mistakes appear under your name in the publication, as well as with the editor's annoyance.**

When checking proofs, it is important to read every word and symbol, however familiar you are with your article. It has been known for drug dosages to be increased to lethal levels by stray decimal points! Remember that the article has been through the hands of the editor and sub-editor, and the graphs or figures have been redrawn by someone else. All sorts of strange things could have happened to your words and ideas, intentionally or accidentally, during these processes.

If the editor has specific queries, these will be marked in the text, usually with a bold question mark and a written question. It is important that you answer these queries and either correct the text, or explain to the editor why it should remain unchanged. A set of internationally recognised symbols are used for correcting proofs (*see* Appendix E), but for a journal article you are usually asked to telephone corrections to the appropriate person rather than send them in on paper. Some important things to remember about correcting proofs are shown in Box 7.1.

Box 7.1:   Dos and don'ts when correcting proofs

DO:
- deal with them immediately
- read through them slowly and carefully
- check boxes, figures and diagrams as well as text
- mark any mistakes clearly so that you don't miss them when talking to the editor
- double-check drug dosages and names, abbreviations and references
- check and deal with any queries marked on the proofs by the editor
- telephone the editor within the time allowed
- contact the editor even if there are no corrections to make

DON'T:
- add new text
- take out or move existing text
- ignore minor mistakes
- miss the deadline for contacting the editor
- assume that your article will be unchanged from the version you sent in
- change the sub-editing (e.g. paragraphing, grammar, etc.)

PUBLICATION (BINGO!)

Once you have phoned in any corrections, or confirmed that there are no corrections to make, you really can sit back and wait for the moment of publication. Your article should appear in the next issue of the journal, and you will usually be sent one or two complimentary copies of the issue in which your article appears. A few publications will also send authors a set of 'offprints' of their article (*see* Chapter 8).

SUMMARY

The writer's work does not end with the completion of an article. There are several stages between submission to a journal and publication when the author's input is essential. These include revising the article if necessary, completing copyright and author's details forms, and correcting page proofs.

WRITE AS YOU READ 7.1

The article that you completed at the end of the last chapter is now ready to be dispatched to your chosen journal. Consult the Guidelines for Contributors to check the format and number of hard copies required, and print off the final versions, or ask your typist for them. Make sure that the final version is also copied to the disk, in ASCII or text form if requested by the journal.

👉 **Don't worry if you suddenly remember that the journal wants double-spacing, or wider margins than you originally thought. So long as you or someone else has the article on a word processor, these things can be corrected at the last minute** (*see* Box 7.2).

Box 7.2:   Clever things you can do on the computer after the article is written

Any word-processing package will allow you to:

- change the margin size
- change the line spacing
- automatically replace a specified word wherever it appears in the text with another word (e.g. 'Drugspeltwrong' with 'Drugspeltright')
- move sections of text
- change the font size
- add page numbers
- add a 'footer', consisting of the title of the article, on each page.

Once your article is ready, you can write the letter to the editor. Remember to include the selling points you discussed with him or her on the telephone, as a reminder. When you actually dispatch your article, in good time to meet your deadline, check its weight at a post office, as it will almost certainly need more than a first-class stamp.

If you receive a letter from the editor in due course requesting revisions, tackle them as soon as possible. Read the reviewer's comments carefully first – you may disagree with some of them and want to discuss them with the editor before undertaking the changes.

👉 **Don't disagree with the reviewer just to save yourself the work of revision. You must have a good argument to make.**

When your revisions are complete, return the article to the editor as soon as possible (aim to get it back to the editor within a couple of weeks). When you receive a letter of acceptance, complete and return the copyright form and author's details form. If the form asks about your availability, mention any holidays when you will not be contactable, so that they do not send you proofs to correct while you are away. You may then have a long wait, but in due course you will receive the page proofs of the article. Read them very carefully and then telephone the editor, whether or not any corrections are needed.

Once you have received your copies of the journal containing your published article, take a few weeks just to enjoy the achievement...then move on to the next chapter.

CHAPTER EIGHT

THINGS TO DO AFTER PUBLICATION

Sometimes an article is published in a professional journal and nothing happens. A copy of the relevant issue is usually sent to the author, and often a cheque follows a few weeks later, but other than that – nothing. Sometimes, however, a whole train of events is set in motion, which often takes the unsuspecting author by surprise. This chapter examines some of the things that may happen after your article is published, and how you might deal with them.

PRACTICAL MATTERS

COPIES

Soon after your article is published, you should receive at least one copy of the issue of the journal in which it features. Some journals send two copies, and others will send a full copy of the relevant journal issue, as well as a number of 'offprints' (*see* Box 8.1).

☞ **Some of the medical newspapers (e.g.** *GP, Doctor*) **do not send any copies to authors. In this case you need to obtain your own copy and, if necessary, photocopy your article.**

It is a good idea to:

- put one copy in your personal professional profile – the research you had to do for the article, and the discipline of writing it, serve as an excellent example of professional development

> **Box 8.1:   Offprints**
>
> 'Offprints' are copies of an article supplied by the journal to the author for their own personal distribution. They consist of the relevant journal pages, printed separately to the rest of the journal, and stapled rather than bound. They look more professional than photocopies or pages cut from a journal, so they are particularly useful for putting in a personal professional profile, and for giving to managers or displaying on notice-boards. Unfortunately, not many nursing journals provide offprints to authors, as they are more expensive to produce than copies of the journal.

- copy the article to anyone who helped with its production (e.g. a friend who read it through for you, or a colleague who supplied an example of good practice)
- copy it to anyone formally involved in the project or work described, if it is that kind of article (e.g. the Chair of a Steering Group, or a course tutor)
- give a copy to your manager, so that they are not taken by surprise when someone else points it out to them – in some units, managers like to keep a file of articles written by staff, or even display them on a notice-board.

PAYMENT

Most of the professional journals do pay authors for published articles. The rate of payment varies considerably from one journal to another, currently ranging from £35 to £200 per 1000 words. The average for the main nursing journals at present is £70–80 per 1000 words.

☞ **The rate of payment offered is usually set out in the commissioning letter (if one has been sent) or in the acceptance letter.**

I have never yet had enough courage to ask an editor, during my conversation with them about a proposed article, how much they will pay for it. Of course, once you have had an article published in a journal and received an acceptance letter, you will know their rate. However, if you are targeting a new journal, you will either have to pluck up the courage to ask – or wait and see!

Once you have received the cheque, it is important to record the payment somewhere, ready to be declared as additional income on your tax return in due course. A sample record sheet for keeping track of articles written and payments received is shown in Appendix G. The first cheque may seem hardly worth the trouble of declaring, but you must because it is the law! Later, it is surprising how quickly those small cheques can add up – writing for publication can bring in very useful extra income (*see* Chapter 9).

QUERIES AND COMMENTS

The first time I was telephoned by an editor with a query from a reader about an article of mine, I was shocked. I had thought that no one would read the article except me and the editor, and possibly some kind friends (who would do so out of a sense of duty, and say appropriately nice things afterwards). Instead, there was an irate woman from somewhere down south, accusing me of misrepresenting some aspect of her area of practice, and demanding redress. I felt terrible. It was like being accused of fraud. As a novice writer, I still felt that somehow it was a mistake that any editor took me seriously enough to publish something I had written. The response from this reader seemed to confirm my worst suspicions – I was a fake and a con artist, and I should be exposed and punished.

The editor was much more blasé. 'At least somebody's reading it,' he said. 'Don't worry about it. There is always somebody who will object, whatever you say.'

However, the editor did require me to produce a response. He published the letter from the reader, together with my reply. And when I stopped beating my breast and read the letter, I found that I could reply to her main points quite easily. It was more a question of emphasis than of fact, and it was easy enough to acknowledge that, and to explain why I had given it the emphasis I had.

👉 **Replies to readers' letters are needed very quickly, as both letters will probably appear in the next issue. Be prepared to write and fax something promptly.**

Not all readers' letters require a reply. Sometimes they simply comment on an article, favourably or otherwise, or add something to the debate on the topic of the article. Editors will publish these without consulting the author of the article, or respond themselves. Only if the writer questions or criticises a specific point will the editor ask the author to provide a reply.

👉 **Don't be surprised if the letters page contains letters about your article which you were not told about in advance. You can either cope with this, or follow my example and give up reading letters pages!**

Apart from letters to the journal, people sometimes write letters directly to the author of an article, and send them via the journal. These will be passed on unopened by the editor. Fortunately, I have found that the letters addressed directly to me, rather than to the editor, tend to be the complimentary ones. However, if they do question the content of the article, you at least have the option of replying directly to the letter writer, rather than having the letter published in the journal. It seems polite to answer these letters unless they are so aggressive in tone as to make further corre-spondence inadvisable. I have not yet received one of the latter type! The only one I nearly didn't reply to was a letter which 'corrected' me on a point of fact about a particular drug, and which the writer had officiously copied to the Secretary of State for Scotland! I wrote back to point out that my information was correct at the time of writing, and the licensing information had changed in the interim. I also suggested that she might like to copy my reply to the Secretary of State.

Some general principles apply to dealing with readers' letters, whether they come directly to you or to the editor.

- Don't be upset by them. Sometimes the tone is so angry, and the complaint so extreme, that you feel personally attacked by it. Remind yourself that the letter writer is only responding to the article, not to you. Reply by talking about the article, or the project/work/topic, rather than yourself.
- Don't be surprised by them. Journals are public property, and will continue to be read for years, as people search back copies for references and information for courses, research or general interest.
- Don't ignore them. If the editor asks you for a reply, you need to produce one. It need only be a couple of lines in length. If someone writes directly to you, you can decide whether to reply, although it is generally advisable to do so.

☞ **It is usually more satisfying to deal with a critical letter by sending off a reply, than by throwing it away and trying to forget it.**

- Complimentary letters are an enormous boost. These are definitely worth keeping in your file with the copies of your articles. After all the hard work that goes into preparing and writing an article, you deserve the appreciation.
- Letters asking for further information really deserve a helpful answer. They are evidence of the usefulness of your article, and should be regarded as a compliment rather than a nuisance.

RESPONDING TO READERS' LETTERS (*see* Box 8.2)

Critical letters usually do one or more of three things:

- question the facts in your article
- take issue with the views expressed in your article
- argue the emphasis or approach taken.

☞ **In preparing your response, bear in mind that the letter writer is not necessarily right – and also that you are not necessarily right all of the time either!**

If the writer questions your facts, you can briefly tell them where you found your information and why you believe it to be correct. This may mean giving a reference, or explaining a point in more detail than appeared in the article. Of course, if they are

---

Box 8.2: Responding to readers' letters

In general, in formulating your reply, aim to be:

- brief
- factual
- polite
- prepared to acknowledge others' points of view.

Example

Thank you for your letter about my article on head lice. I agree with you that the electric lice comb can be a valuable tool for parents. I omitted discussion of the full range of resources available, as the main focus of the article was the controversy about chemical treatments. However, I shall certainly include a full resource list in any reprints of this article.

Try not to be:

- defensive
- offensive
- didactic.

Example

Thank you for your letter pointing out the mistakes and omissions in my article on head lice. You clearly are not aware that many research articles dispute the usefulness of the electric lice comb (Smith, 1998, Jones, 1997, Cobbley et al., 1999, inter alia). As a member of a profession that practices evidence-based care, it would be irresponsible to promote the use of this tool on such an uncertain evidence base.

---

right to question the fact, because there is an error in the article, acknowledge it gracefully, thank them for bringing it to your attention, and say that you will let the editor know about the error. Avoiding such admissions is one of the reasons why it is important to use good references and information when writing the article, and a fine-tooth comb when proof-reading! If the writer takes issue with your opinions, your answer can be very short and simple. You should acknowledge that there are other points of view, but point out that you have simply expressed your own. If you wish, you can go on to justify your stance, but you may well feel that you do not want to engage in such a debate.

If the writer argues with the approach or emphasis that you used, you can adopt much the same approach in your reply. You appreciate their taking the trouble to respond to the article, but you were bringing your own perspective to it. Another writer could have used a different approach. Again, you might want to explain why the purpose of your article required the approach you used – or you might not.

REPRINTS

Some time after your article has been printed, you may be informed by the journal that they intend to reprint your article, either in one of their related journals (*see* Box 8.3), or as a special educational booklet, for example.

Box 8.3:   Some examples of related journals

Nursing Standard
    Primary Health Care
    Elderly Care
    Emergency Nurse
    Nursing Management
    ...and others

Nursing Times
    Community Nurse
    NT Research
    ...and others

Community Practitioners' and Health Visitors' Association
    Community Practitioner
    Mental Health Nursing

☛ **Remember, the journal owns the copyright to your article, so they do not need your permission to reprint your article.**

Sometimes you will be asked to check the article prior to reprinting, to ensure that the information that it contains is still current, and that there are no essential additions to make. This is a valuable opportunity to put right any errors made in the original (*see* Box 8.4), but not generally to rewrite large sections of the article. If the article is reprinted in a related journal that targets a different readership, you may be asked to adapt your article slightly for the new journal. For example, an article that I wrote on tuberculosis, for *Nursing Standard*'s continuing education series, was reprinted in two of that journal's sister publications, *Emergency Nurse* and *Primary Health Care*. To adapt it for these different outlets, I had to:

●   make some slight changes in the section on the nurse's role in the care of patients with tuberculosis, since this is clearly different in Accident and Emergency departments and in the community

- change one of the case study-based questions in the assessment to reflect the type of patient who would be familiar to nurses reading these journals.

Box 8.4:   Correcting for reprinting – urinalysis

I wrote an article on urinalysis as part of an educational series. A section of the article was concerned with *in-vitro* testing of urine using 'dip-stick' testing strips. I used the *MIMS*, the *British National Formulary* and some manufacturers' materials for information on testing strips.

   After the article was published, I received a letter from a representative of one of the manufacturers of testing strips. He complimented me on using the correct term ('strips' rather than 'stix', which was the name used by the rival manufacturer), but pointed out some subtle differences between the usage and reading of the different makes of strips, which I had failed to mention in the article.

   I wrote back and thanked him for the information, assuring him that I would ensure that future printings included the correct information. Unfortunately, the article was reprinted in a sister journal without my prior knowledge, and all the same inaccuracies were repeated. This time I had to write to the manufacturers to apologise.

Most publications offer a payment of half the original sum for reprinting an article without amendments, and more if some revision work has to be carried out by the author.

CONTACTS

It is worth repeating that the professional journals are the public property of the profession as a whole, and we should not be surprised that articles in them are read, reread, referenced, researched and regurgitated for years after their original publication. Once you have an article published in a journal, your name is attached to it and to the topic forever. People will make contact with the authors of articles they have read, usually by writing to the journal that published the article, for a variety of different reasons. I have had contacts from people:

- asking for more information on a project described in an article
- asking for updated information on the results of studies or outcomes of projects
- thanking me for providing them with reference material for course assignments
- asking for advice on implementing similar initiatives in their area
- asking me to speak to special interest groups
- inviting me to join national reference groups
- inviting me to contribute to other planned publications.

As far as possible, I try to respond positively to such approaches. Of course, it may not be possible for you to speak at a conference, or to arrange a visit to a particular service which was the topic of your article, but there is usually someone else with whom the enquirer can be put in contact. These approaches from readers really are compliments, and not to respond in a helpful way would be like accepting a bouquet without even saying thank you.

SUMMARY

Authors of articles in nursing journals may be contacted by readers following publication, either directly or via the letters page of the journal. If the editor asks for a reply to publish with a reader's letter, it is essential that it is provided quickly. A brief explanation is usually all that is required. Responses made directly to the letter writer should generally be brief, polite and objective. At later stages, authors may be asked to review their article prior to reprinting. This is an opportunity to put right any inaccuracies in the first version that may have been brought to light. In addition, writers are sometimes contacted by readers for further information, or with invitations to speak to groups or write for other publications. Such approaches are almost invariably complimentary, and deserve a positive response.

CHAPTER NINE

HOW TO BE A REGULAR

Why, you might wonder, after all that work to produce an article and see it through to publication, should anyone want to repeat the experience regularly? There are many reasons to keep writing:

- for the fame – it is undoubtedly gratifying to see your name in print on a piece of work of which you are proud and, in my experience, this pleasure does not diminish over the years. It is also rewarding to be contacted by people to say that they have referenced your work in their assignment or their thesis, or to be introduced at a meeting and have people say 'Oh, I saw your article...'. You know you have achieved your ambition to be a regular contributor to the journals when you can answer that with the question 'Which one?'
- for the money – no one will ever retire on the money paid by the nursing journals for articles, or even on the royalties from a textbook. However, it is entirely possible to earn a few thousand pounds a year if you can produce articles efficiently, so regular writing can fund holidays, or make some impact on the cost of putting a child through university.
- for the professional credibility – in some areas of practice, publishing in the professional journals is considered to be essential. If you want to work in a university department of health or nursing, publication is a real boost to your job application. Once there, you will be expected to continue to publish. If you are interested in research, you will find that most job advertisements ask for a record of research and publication.

☞ **Even though jobs in research may require publications related to research, publications of any sort are a good start, and a way to build up confidence and expertise.**

- for professional advancement – even if you do not aspire to a job which requires you to publish, it is helpful to any nursing career to have published articles on your area of practice. The background research and reading undertaken before writing, and the discipline of producing a structured and coherent account, provide an excellent learning experience for the writer. This is one of the reasons why the production of any article should be recorded in your personal professional profile, and can contribute to meeting the requirements of the post-registration education and practice (PREP) programme. Such personal learning can only help to prepare you for moving on in your career. In addition, a list of publications makes your CV stand out from many others, and so can positively enhance your prospects of getting a job.
- for the other opportunities – if you write regularly in the professional journals, you will find that many other opportunities come your way. You may be asked to write more articles or series, to speak to special interest groups, to speak at a conference or training day, to write a training manual or educational materials, or to sit on local, regional or national committees relevant to your area of practice. If you want to develop and broaden your career, writing regularly for the nursing journals is a very good way to do so.

☞ **If your name appears on many articles related to a particular area of practice (which may be as broad as 'primary care' or as specific as 'continence'), you will quickly become regarded as an expert in that area.**

GROUND RULES

If you want to write regularly for the nursing press, you can. If you have had one article published, you can do it again – and again and again. All it takes is a systematic approach, and the commitment of some time.

☞ **You don't have to be 'better' than everyone else to be published regularly. Some of what is published in the nursing press is decidedly average, but remember that the editors have their pages to fill!**

So you don't have to be a clinical whiz-kid, or an academic high-flyer, to feature regularly in the journals, but you do have to be:

- professional about your writing
- consistent in the quality of your writing
- reliable in relation to delivery, deadlines, dealing with queries, etc.
- resilient when challenged or criticised
- committed to spending the necessary time and effort on your writing.

STARTING OUT

Whatever types of articles you think you may want to write, there are some simple steps to take in order to prepare (*see* Box 9.1). The reading and analysis of other articles should continue throughout your writing career, as there are always new ideas, new formats and new opportunities to discover in different publications. Always writing the same kind of article, in the same style, makes writing much easier and quicker – but it can also make it stale and tedious, and sooner or later editors will start looking for something different.

Box 9.1: Preparation for regular writing

To prepare for writing regularly:

- regularly read a variety of articles, using different styles, in different journals
- systematically assess the styles, formats and approaches used in other writers' articles
- be prepared to start by writing shorter, stand-alone articles rather than series
- develop an eye and ear for subjects, stories, anecdotes, achievements and initiatives which could provide material for articles
- organise a space for writing, with a file for correspondence with editors, and a book for recording income and expenses (*see* Appendix G).

It is also essential, when you start to write regularly, to assemble some information resources which you can access quickly and easily as you plan and write your articles. These could include:

- files of relevant articles and a filing system (*see* Box 9.2)
- some essential reference books (*see* Box 9.3)
- other relevant books (e.g. on your clinical topic or your area of practice)
- a full set of the UKCC booklets (e.g. on Code of Conduct, Scope of Professional Practice, record-keeping), which you will refer to often
- getting connected to the Internet and the World Wide Web (*see* Appendix F)
- membership of a local nursing, medical or health studies library, as an external member if necessary

☞ **Do not be put off by the difficulty of joining a library if you are not on a course, or if you work in an area such as general practice. You *must* have access to all the latest journals, and to a wide range of books.**

- subscriptions to the one or two most relevant journals – these might be one

---

Box 9.2:   Filing systems

Everyone has their own method of filing, but to save time and prevent interruption of the flow of your writing, you need some kind of system for keeping articles, leaflets, booklets, etc., which you may consult when you are writing an article.

   As an example, my main area of professional expertise is primary care. The different aspects of primary care on which I write most often are filed under subheadings so that I can track down relevant reference material quickly and reliably:

Primary Care
    Policy
    Nursing
            Practice nursing
                    Clinical
                    Education
            Health visiting
            District nursing
            Primary health care teams
    Quality
            In nursing
            In general practice
    Primary care groups
            Policy documents
            Articles
            Primary care trusts
    Clinical
            Immunisation
            Women's health
            Heart disease
            Asthma

---

general and one specialist journal in your area of nursing. You can offset these subscriptions as expenses against your income from writing when you complete your Inland Revenue self-assessment form

- a list of relevant web sites on which you will find copies of relevant policy documents, news about professional developments, reviews of research evidence, etc. (*see* Box 9.4).

Obtaining these resources need not be an expensive undertaking. For example, a good way to obtain newly published textbooks is to offer to review them for a professional

---

Box 9.3: Essential reference books

Some of the books and leaflets I have found essential in writing a range of articles include:

- a *Dictionary of Nursing*
- a *British National Formulary*
- all of the UKCC leaflets on professional matters
- a good anatomy and physiology text
- the *Effective Care Bulletins* from the University of York Centre for Reviews and Dissemination
- major policy reports and documents as they are published (e.g. '*The New NHS*' White Paper, '*Our Healthier Nation*' Green Paper, the consultation on the Strategy for Nursing, Midwifery and Health Visiting).

Box 9.4:   Some useful web sites for nursing and health information

- Nurse WWW Information Service: http://medweb/bham.ac.uk/nursing
- The Department of Health Home Page:
     http://www.open.gov.uk/doh/dhhome.htm
- Health Services Research Super Highway:
     http://www.york.ac.uk/– jmm7/places.htm
- Healthgate: http://www.healthgate.com
- Centre for Evidence-Based Medicine: http://cebm.jr2.ox.ac.uk
- Clinical Guidelines Index:
     http://www.healthcentre.org.uk/hc/library/guidelines/htm
- Patient Information: http://www.rcgp.org.uk/faculty/severn/frames.htm
- World Health Organisation: http://www.who.ch

---

journal. Editors often have great difficulty in finding people who are willing to write book reviews (which are usually only 100–300 words each), and they are usually very pleased to have an offer from someone with relevant expertise. You will be sent a copy of the book, sometimes before it appears on the bookshop shelves, with some guidance about the type of information to be included in the review. Once the review is completed, you are free to keep the book.

A good source of UKCC leaflets is the local nursing library, which often has shelves full of the leaflets, and invites you to take them away. If you get such an opportunity, take the full set – you may not think that you need to know the Midwives Rules if you work in coronary care, but you never know what you will be writing about next!

A good place to find a range of useful information is the big national nursing conferences. In the exhibition hall you will often find stands for the UKCC, the English National Board, the Department of Health, the Health Education Authority and the professional associations. All of these provide free copies of books, leaflets and monographs which are invaluable for background to articles, key facts and statistics. Use that free carrier bag and take away as much as you can carry.

Conference exhibitions also often include voluntary organisations related to health care, alternative therapy practitioners, charities and special interest groups, which provide leaflets and information as well as contacts. These are very useful for giving a wider perspective to articles, suggesting a different approach or a different subject altogether.

For example, if you usually write about surgical nursing, a walk around the stands at an exhibition might give you several new ideas.

- The Association for the Victims of Medical Accidents might suggest a piece on the support available for patients whose surgery is not as successful as they hoped.
- An aromatherapy practitioner might talk enthusiastically about the pain and stress-relieving properties of essential oils, and lead you to plan an article describing the evidence for the effectiveness of non-pharmaceutical methods of post-operative pain relief.
- The Health Education Authority's display of glossy patient information leaflets might remind you of the shortage of good leaflets on specialised surgery, and lead you to write about the effect of good pre-operative information on patients' experience of surgery.

Other places where you can collect useful information and make contacts are study days and courses. Get into the habit of collecting books, handouts, leaflets and articles, but also ensure that you have some kind of filing system so that you can track down the piece you require when you need it!

REGULAR WRITING: THE OPTIONS

There are three main forms of regular writing for professional journals:

- regular, stand-alone pieces
- series
- regular columns.

The stand-alone pieces may be clinical or professional articles, opinion or comment articles, or shorter pieces such as book reviews.

CLINICAL/PROFESSIONAL ARTICLES

For the clinical or professional articles, there are two approaches to writing regularly. You can either write as an expert, in one or a few clearly defined areas of practice (e.g. continence, nurse prescribing or health screening); or you can make yourself a generalist, writing about a wide range of topics, probably in less depth and detail. The advantages and disadvantages of both of these approaches are shown in Box 9.5.

	Box 9.5: Some of the advantages and disadvantages of writing as a specialist or generalist	
	Advantages	**Disadvantages**
Specialist/ expert	You can concentrate your reading in one subject area There will be less competition from other writers You can combine learning for your 'day job' with research for your writing You will need fewer reference resources It is easier to keep up with new developments in one area You will build a reputation more quickly	You may be restricted to fewer journals Your reputation will be linked to one topic only You may get bored with the subject
Generalist	You have many more topics to write about You will not be associated with one topic in editors' minds The variety is more interesting and more challenging You have a wider range of journals to target You will learn about a range of topics	You will need much more reference material You will not be regarded as an expert in any area You may need to do more research

Finding topics to write about should not be difficult, even if you are an expert in a very specialised topic. To find ideas:

- keep up to date with news on policies, new drugs or treatments reported in the nursing press, which could form the focus of an article
- use your professional networks and talk to people working in the same, similar or related areas of practice, to find out about their experiences and ideas
- make new contacts whenever you can – someone you meet at a conference, or the author of an article in your area of practice, could be approached for a discussion which leads to a new angle on the topic
- try to see all relevant policy documents, either through your manager or nursing library, or by obtaining your own copy, as you may notice something relevant to your area of practice.

If you are a generalist, identify some broad areas in which you feel you can write (e.g. 'acute care', 'children's nursing' or 'education'). Then do all the things suggested above, but with a very broad perspective. Aim to be an opportunist – almost anything can be the starting point for an article if you are ready to write one.

SOME EXAMPLES

A writer specialising in the topic of wound care gives a presentation to practice nurses about the management of leg ulcers. This simple activity, part of his or her everyday practice, could lead to a whole range of articles:

- an opinion piece about the way in which conditions perceived as 'unglamorous' are unpopular with nurses, for a general nursing publication
- a general article about the treatment of leg ulcers, for a practice nurse journal
- a technical article about the use of brachial pressure index measurement for differentiating ulcers of venous and arterial origin, for a professional nursing journal
- a descriptive piece on the costs and impact of a specialist nurse in a leg ulcer clinic, for a management publication
- a skill-sharing article on preparing presentations, for a student nurse supplement.

A generalist writer, sitting in the audience of the same leg ulcer study day, might come away with a completely different set of ideas for articles:

- a discussion piece about the relative effectiveness of doctors and nurses as teachers of nurses, for a general nursing journal
- an opinion piece about the hidden reasons people have for attending study days on particular topics, for a general publication
- a skills-sharing piece about reflecting on educational events in order to complete personal professional profiles, for a professional nursing journal

- a review of the evidence about effective teaching strategies for adult learners, for an educational journal.

☞ **It is useful to get into the habit of writing down your ideas as they occur to you, so that when you are ready to plan your article, you have the topic already defined.**

OPINION ARTICLES

Opinion pieces are a good way to start writing regularly. There is always something happening in nursing or healthcare which is worthy of comment, and the editors of weekly publications in particular are often keen to have topical opinion pieces to fill designated pages. By writing regularly, you soon develop a style which makes the writing relatively quick and easy, and builds a reputation for you with the journal and its readers.

Unlike clinical pieces, opinion pieces usually need to be:

- topical – written within days or weeks of an event, not months afterwards
- original – they are unlikely to be published if they merely repeat a common opinion
- distinctive – your 'voice' (the combination of your writing style and your views) should come through clearly.

☞ **Just because they are not clinical articles, opinion pieces do not need any less attention to good spelling, grammar and presentation. You need to be as professional and reliable in your dealings with the journal as you would if you were submitting any other article.**

The best way to develop your 'voice' and establish yourself is to make a start. Read the weekly journals' opinion pages, and see what kind of word length they publish, and on what type of topic. As a quick response to events or ideas is essential in opinion pieces, this is one time when you may not need to telephone the editor before writing. If you do, just check that they would be interested in a piece on the topic. There is no need to discuss it in much detail, and there is a positive advantage to your opinion arriving fresh on the editor's desk.

☞ **Aim to write one piece every few weeks, for the same journal. This will help you to develop your voice and speed up your writing, as well as bringing your name to the editor's attention.**

How do you keep finding topics about which to write opinion pieces? Try:

- reading the news and analysis pages for incidents or announcements which trigger comment ('Bogus nurse worked for 3 years...')

- reading the daily newspapers for health-related stories which could form a background
- checking lists of anniversaries, births and deaths, and famous events, for something you could comment on
- looking at recent opinion pieces and taking a different perspective on the same topic
- making unusual connections between nursing and events apparently unrelated to the profession.

☞ **Opinion pieces do not have to contain startling insights or profound messages. They just have to give an opinion, clearly and distinctively, for others to read and perhaps comment on.**

A word of warning should be given here. It is intoxicating to develop a recognisable voice, and to find yourself published regularly and have people commenting to you about your articles. It is easy to be carried away by success, and to write unwisely. As an old pro who has made all the mistakes, I can only offer some ground rules for sensible writing in this field (*see* Box 9.6), which you will undoubtedly want to break at regular intervals. There is a balance to be found between 'safe' writing which is emasculated and unchallenging, and taking risks which may bring very unpleasant censure. None of us treads the middle path successfully all of the time!

☞ **It is not the editor's job to save you from the consequences of any extreme opinions or criticisms in your article – they may publish them simply in order to generate debate and controversy.**

SAME JOURNAL OR DIFFERENT JOURNALS?

Once you begin to write regularly, you will have to decide whether to keep targeting the same journal, or to spread your efforts across a number of different publications. The pros and cons of each approach are shown in Box 9.7. If you find time to write fairly quickly, and are able to produce an article a month (or more), it is likely that you will have to target a range of journals. No single publication will be able to use all of your material at that rate. In general, the diversity of opportunity, the discipline of matching different styles and requirements, and the sheer professional challenge make it infinitely preferable to have as broad a range of target publications as possible.

NEXT STEPS

Both opinion pieces and clinical or professional articles, published regularly under your name in one or more professional journals, can lead to further offers of work.

Box 9.6:   Some ideal ground rules for opinion pieces

- Avoid criticising named institutions or individuals.
- Acknowledge that there are different views to your own.
- Do not express racist, sexist or similar sentiments.
- Do not use the first person ('I') too often.
- Avoid ranting or whinging.
- Use humour to soften criticism.

Box 9.7:   Pros and cons of writing for different journals

Should you concentrate on targeting one journal, or write for as wide a variety as possible?

	Advantages	**Disadvantages**
One journal	You will build a relationship with the editor more quickly Your name will quickly become known to their readers Knowing the journal's style and approach will save time in planning and writing	You are limited to the number of articles they can take You will only gain experience of writing in one style You are limited to the topics covered by that journal
Lots of journals	You will be able to write in different styles You will have a wider range of topics to write about You will become known to a range of editors You can have more articles published You are more likely to be commissioned to do other work	You have to build relationships with many different editors You need to adapt your writing style and approach to each journal's needs

---

This is that magical moment when, instead of you always asking someone else to consider publishing your article, someone asks you if you will consider writing an article for them! Take time out to celebrate. I still have two faded congratulations cards that were sent to me when I was asked to write my first regular column, in *Nursing Standard*. They bring back all the excitement of the time when I first felt I was succeeding at something I had always wanted to do.

WRITING FOR A SERIES

The logical next step to writing regular stand-alone articles is to write a series. You might start by contributing one or more articles to an existing series, such as the formal, distance-learning articles which appear in the weekly nursing press, or by suggesting a new series to an editor.

☞ **You will probably need a track record of one-off publications before an editor will risk accepting a series from you. They need to be sure that you can write, and that you can deliver!**

If you want to contribute to an existing series, you must be very familiar with it before you discuss it with the editor. Make sure that you know the types of articles included, the intervals at which they appear, and the topics they have already covered. When you speak to the editor:

- be prepared for the fact that they may already have commissioned all of the articles they need for the series
- have a list of your previous published articles ready to demonstrate that you can write publishable material, to deadlines and pre-arranged word lengths
- be prepared to match your style or approach to that of the rest of the series – you may need not only clinical knowledge of the topic, but the ability to write test questions or provide student learning activities as well
- have some ideas for topics that you could contribute to the series – try to have at least two or three, as some topics may already have been commissioned
- be prepared for the editor to suggest a completely different topic – there may be a topic which needs to be covered and that does not currently have an author
- do not agree to write about something unless you are sure you know (or can find out) enough about the subject – in other words, do not agree just for the sake of being published, as your reputation will suffer if you have to pull out later.

If you are going to suggest a new series, make sure that you can justify the number of articles to be included and explain why the topics could not be handled in one article. It is important to avoid the impression that a series is simply more profitable than a single article!

From the editor's point of view, accepting a series means committing page space for weeks or months (depending on the frequency of publication and the number of articles in the series), and reducing the opportunities to take more topical material.

For ideas for a series, look at some of the existing series in the journals you might target. There might be a series of interesting cases, a revision series on basic nursing topics, or a series about nurses with unusual jobs, or older nurses, or nurses from a particular background. It is pointless to copy an existing idea – editors are always looking for a new twist or a fresh approach. However, existing series can provide a starting point for some lateral thinking. If someone has produced a series about 'high-flyers' in nursing, what about a series on 'bedside' nurses, who have spent 20–30 years in direct patient care? If the topic of 'older nurses' has already been covered, is there scope for a series on the new cadet nurse schemes being restarted in some areas? Some of your ideas will make series, while others will not have the scope and will end up as a single article. Write the single article while you think some more about your series!

When planning a series, it is important for there to be a clear and logical link between the articles. There are numerous ways to make such a link:

- by area of practice (e.g. series about different complementary therapies)
- by patient group (e.g. series on men's health)
- by underpinning policy (e.g. articles on each of the four key areas of 'Our Healthier Nation')
- by educational purpose (e.g. articles on key professional guidelines).

The other important aspect of planning a series is time-scale. If the series is to run weekly for 4 weeks, you will have to deliver all four articles either at the same time, or in very quick succession. Even if the series is for a monthly publication, the editor is likely to want the first couple of articles at the same time, with the others on short deadlines thereafter. Look ahead at your calendar to check that you don't have holidays, major life events or other impediments which may stop you delivering four, five or six articles within a short space of time.

☞ **Be absolutely sure that you have time to write the series before you offer it to anyone!**

WRITING A REGULAR COLUMN

This is something which, generally speaking, you wait to be invited to do. Editors need to be familiar with your name and your style, and convinced of your profession-alism and reliability, before they risk commissioning you for a regular column. After all, a column is a form of never-ending series! There are not many such columns in the nursing press, and, where they do exist, they may be occupied by the same incumbent for years. The best preparation for an invitation to write a column is:

- to write regularly for a number of journals
- to develop different styles and use them in a range of different types of article

- to deal professionally and personally with editors
- to be 100% reliable
- to be patient!

However, you should keep an eye out for opportunities. I acquired one of my regular columns because the journal advertised that its present columnist was giving up for personal reasons, and invited readers to volunteer to take her place. I then had to produce three full columns, and a plan for 6 months' more columns, to convince the editor that I could take on the task. The commission is renewed on an annual basis, if both the editor and I decide that this is what we want to do.

It is always possible that an unsolicited idea for a regular column will be accepted. Work out the idea in detail before discussing it with the editor, and be prepared to submit two or three sample columns in advance of a decision.

CONTENT OF THE COLUMN

The content of a regular column published under the author's name is usually a personal perspective on a topical professional issue. Often this is provided by an expert in the journal's field, in which case you would need to be able to convince the editor that you have the right qualifications or experience, as well as the writing ability, to take on such a column. However, there are several alternatives to the 'expert's perspective':

- a humorous perspective (this will be discussed in more detail in the next chapter)
- an 'alternative' perspective – this is any off-beat, 'sideways' look at the topic, for which you will need to convince the editor that you can continue to produce such slants over a long period of time
- a 'practitioner's' perspective – this type of column takes the 'ordinary nurse' viewpoint, and you need to be able to claim honestly that you are such an ordinary nurse, but with added professionalism, reliability and writing ability, of course!

Another form of regular column is the diary. It is a form which has been used fairly frequently in the past, and because it is not original, it needs to come from an unusual angle to be worth publishing. 'The diary of a student nurse' is not likely to catch an editor's attention, but the diary of a cadet might, because cadet nursing is an old idea which has been revived, and readers could be interested in how it works in today's hospitals. Similarly, the diary of the first 'nurse consultant' would be more enticing than that of a newly qualified staff nurse.

☛ **Remember that the rewards of a regular income and a modest degree of fame have to be balanced against the relentless demands of regular deadlines and the need to produce an endless stream of new ideas.**

Anonymous columns

If the aim is to see your name at the top of a column, you may be disappointed. Quite a few of the regular columns in the professional press have a pseudonym, or simply a title, rather than the author's name. Examples are 'Detritus' and 'Backbite' in *Practice Nurse*, 'Synapse' and the erstwhile 'Sister Plume' in *Nursing Times*, the former 'Sister Susie' in *Nursing Standard*, and 'Gadfly' and 'Monitor' in the *Health Service Journal*.

The advantage of writing in this way is that you can be deliberately cynical, provocative, outspoken or otherwise challenging, without compromising your day-to-day credibility with your colleagues or employer. Having written three of the anonymous columns cited above, I find this freedom enormously entertaining. I also think that it is important that readers can be challenged in this way, so that the entirely appropriate and worthy professionalism of the rest of the journal is balanced by some personal views and opinions which can spark healthy debate, even if it ends in disagreement.

OTHER REGULAR FEATURES

Falling somewhere between the short series and the regular column are other forms of the regularly commissioned feature. These include:

- book reviews
- web site reviews
- quizzes and other puzzles
- television or media reviews
- 'journal scans'.

These are ideal ways to begin writing regularly, and to demonstrate your reliability and 'sticking power'. It is always worth discussing ideas for this type of feature with an editor. In my experience, editors are always looking for book reviewers in particular, and for ideas for something a little different to fill small sections on these pages. Although they may sound routine, these types of feature do not have to be boring. It is perfectly possible to write challenging and interesting book reviews, or zany and humorous quizzes. In fact, the more distinctive your voice in these pieces, the more likely you are to be asked to write more or different articles.

SUMMARY

Anyone who has had an article published in a professional journal can become a regular writer if they are prepared to put time and effort into developing their writing. Writing articles regularly can lead to whole series, regular features or even regular columns being published. Smaller features such as book reviews and quizzes can be a useful way to establish writing credibility, and to forge relationships with editors.

CHAPTER TEN

How to be funny

Writing 'funny' material for the professional press does not necessarily mean provoking belly laughs from the readers. In this context, it means any material which is intended to be light-hearted, humorous or satirical. And while personal style – often the source of the humour – has to be developed by the writer, there are some useful tips about approaches to humorous writing which can be learned.

Why humorous writing?

Some people would argue that there is no place in a serious professional journal for humorous writing. In some of the more academic publications, any trace of light-heartedness is limited to the occasional witticism in the editorial. However, there are a number of justifications for using humour in the professional press:

- it can help learning, by presenting information in a form which people are more likely to read (*see* Box 10.1)
- it can make challenges to the *status quo*, to 'received wisdom' or make new ideas more palatable
- it can bring a fresh perspective to issues which might otherwise become so earnest and narrowly focused that some of their meaning would be lost
- it can simply amuse and entertain professionals whose working lives are generally busy and stressful, and sometimes traumatic.

Opportunities for humorous writing

It is surprising how many opportunities there are for humorous writing in the nursing and other professional publications. The weekly magazines *Nursing Standard*

Box 10.1:   Humour as learning

This quiz appeared in *Nursing Standard*, and although its main aim was to amuse, it was also educational. The NHS reforms were not well understood by many nurses, and answer (a) to each question is actually correct. A few of the questions are shown here:

What is the effect of the 'internal market'?
  (a)   Separation of the purchaser and provider functions in healthcare
  (b)   Changing the names of hospitals to trusts
  (c)   Setting up craft stalls in hospital reception areas
  (d)   Opening up intimate examinations to competitive tender

Which of the following is a provider organisation?
  (a)   A hospital trust
  (b)   The National Trust
  (c)   A surgical truss
  (d)   Sainsburys

What is a finished consultant episode?
  (a)   A measure of hospital activity used in contracts
  (b)   A measure of psychiatric disease in hospital specialists
  (c)   A professional conduct hearing for doctors
  (d)   The bit where Julian leaves *Casualty*

What is BS5750?
  (a)   An accreditation of quality
  (b)   A very high blood sugar reading
  (c)   A form of mad cow disease
  (d)   The last flight out to the Bahamas

Reproduced with permission from *Nursing Standard*
Cook R (1995) Round the reforms. *Nursing Standard* **10**: 35.

---

and *Nursing Times* both carry regular columns, opinion pieces, personal perspective pieces and 'stand-alone' articles in which humour is a major feature. Other publications have at least a regular page or feature written in a light-hearted style, designed to entertain, inform, or both. Some examples are the 'Backbite' feature in *Practice Nurse*, and 'Gadfly' and 'Monitor' in the *Health Service Journal*.

Good humorous writing is probably a lot less common than good articles in more conventional styles, so the target market is wider than just the nursing journals. Editors from many different professional sectors are willing to look at humorous writing, because it is the ability to write entertainingly, rather than any clinical expertise, which counts. There are many common features of health, health services, the professions and the patients that they serve, which make it possible for a doctor to write light pieces for nursing journals, nurses to write for management journals, and so on (*see* Box 10.2 for some examples). In fact, the medical press seems to have a much more robust attitude to humour, and welcomes all kinds of satirical and humorous writing.

Box 10.2: Crossing the professional boundaries with humour

Examples of humorous articles I have had published in non-nursing journals:

Topic	Publication
Clinical governance	*Doctor*
Fundholding	*Management in General Practice*
GP trainees	*General Practitioner*
Blood donation	The *Guardian*
Travel vaccination	The *Guardian*
Practice nursing	*American Journal of Nursing*

Of course, there are journals which do not run humorous columns or articles. The research journals and some of the publications at the more serious end of the nursing scale are not fertile ground for humorous writers.

☞ **Do not send funny articles to these journals 'on spec', as you will only irritate the editor and ruin your reputation.**

GETTING STARTED IN GENERAL

It is very helpful to read everything you can that has been written in this vein by other people and published in professional journals, or in compilation form in books. Their approaches, formats, topics and individual 'voices' can all provide inspiration and education, as well as a pragmatic guide to what editors publish.

☞ **You will not succeed by deliberately imitating other humorous writers, but you may well succeed by adapting, developing and reinventing your own ways of writing to produce fresh, personal, funny pieces.**

This is what makes this form of writing so rewarding. As well as entertaining people, and all the fun of having people compliment you on that, you are constantly challenged to be creative, innovative and daring in the way that you write, as well as in what you say.

Of course, it helps to read funny writing published in other places as well, such as novels, newspaper columns, magazine features, posters and books. There is something to be learned from every piece of humorous writing about what works well and what is not so successful, depending on the reader's sense of humour and experiences, as well as formats and phraseology. I once saw a poster in a jeans shop headed 'Ten ways to tell you're the village psychopath', followed by a list of clues (such as laughing at horror videos). This gave me an idea for a whole series of pieces under the heading 'Ten ways to tell...' (*see* Box 10.3 for an example from this series).

Box 10.3:   'Ten ways to tell...'

The idea for this format came from a poster I noticed on a shopping trip.

10 ways to tell ... you'd be great at research

1   You know what 'CINAHL' stands for
2   You refer to your friends as '*et al.*'
3   You list references for job applications in alphabetical order by surname
4   You put references on your postcards: 'hotel not as described in brochure (SunHols, 1998)'
5   When your friends take drugs at parties, you insist on organising a control group
6   Then you write it up for publication
7   Your friends think you're boring
8   Your mother thinks you're boring
9   You can't choose a sandwich without carrying out a literature search first
10 You wouldn't have come into nursing in the days before you could wear a gown at your graduation

---

It is important to remember that there is no right or wrong way to write humorously. Whatever style or approach you adopt for a piece, some people will find it hilarious while others will be completely unmoved, or even irritated. This applies to all of the famous newspaper columnists and comic novelists, as well as to the rest of us.

☞ **Humorous writing is much more risky than other writing, in which you are only using words as a tool to describe something. In humorous writing you are also saying 'listen to this, this is funny'.**

GETTING STARTED FOR YOURSELF

Writing humorous pieces requires much the same preparation and research work as writing any other article. The essential first steps are basically the same, although the way you approach them may be different.

- Identify your topic.
- Define your topic.
- Know your journal.
- Approach the editor.

Identifying your topic means pinning down that fleeting idea for a funny article. Ideas for humorous writing do not usually arrive as logically as those for more conventional articles. Instead of thinking 'I must write up this brilliant project we've got going', or 'Today's students obviously need a basic understanding of the NHS reforms', you are more likely to have had a passing thought on a topic, which you vaguely think could be turned into something amusing. Perhaps you had your first experience of working in the community, and you felt like an alien from another planet. Or a patient told you about giving birth to twins in the days before scans and other antenatal scrutiny, and how the doctor delivering her fainted when he saw the second head emerging. In each case, it crossed your mind that you could make a funny piece out of it. The important thing at this point is to write down the idea, before it disappears into the daily round and is lost forever. The encounters which give rise to such ideas are serendipitous, chance occurrences which are never repeated, unlike the projects you work with daily, or repeated exposure to people with educational needs.

 It may sound corny and pretentious to carry a notebook for such ideas, but it does help – and as each idea nets you a cheque for a published article, you find you can live with being corny and pretentious!

Having captured your idea, you need to define your 'angle' on the topic in a little more detail. For humorous writing, this also means choosing the approach that you will take to the piece. Again, this is a slightly different process to defining your topic for a 'straight' article, which involved sitting down to plan, and narrowing the focus to define exactly what aspect of the topic you were going to deal with, what the purpose was, and the target readership. For a humorous piece it is usually a more protracted process, in which you let the idea mature and ferment in your mind until you know the angle you will take.

Take the first of the examples above, namely working in the community for the first time. There are many different ways to develop this idea. For example, you could:

- make it a general piece about nurses coping with changes of clinical area, using all your experience of moving between wards, hospitals, days and nights, etc.
- focus on the culture shock of moving from 'inside hospital' to 'outside hospital'
- compare the reality of the community with the portrayal of community nursing on the television
- compare the different characteristics of hospital and community nurses.

Which of these angles – or others – you decide on will depend on a combination of many internal and external factors (*see* Box 10.4).

Box 10.4:   Factors affecting choice of topic

Internal factors	**External factors**
Your experiences	What has already been written
Your fund of stories and anecdotes	What people around you find amusing
Your interests and preferences	The target readership
Your contacts	The journal you are targeting
Your information resources	Current affairs in nursing
Your job/position/colleagues	

After choosing your angle, you need to decide on the approach. The approach to a 'straight' clinical or professional article is usually obvious. Most of these articles are written as plain narrative, with subheadings and charts, diagrams or figures to break up the text and add interest. For a humorous piece, there are many more choices.

Your reading of other people's humorous articles in a variety of publications will probably have demonstrated at least four different approaches:

- narrative – plain text that tells stories, expresses opinions or describes things in a humorous way
- perspective pieces – the text is often more colourful, written in the first person (using 'I'), and may take a deliberately provocative tone (some regular columns use this approach)
- spoof items – these copy the techniques used for serious pieces, but use them for unusual topics – formats commonly used in this way include multiple-choice questions and quizzes (*see* Box 10.1)
- satire – this approach uses a 'parallel reality' to convey a message. The piece appears to be written 'straight', but both the message and the humour are in the comparison of the situation being described with the way the reader knows the world to be. It is important that the humour is never acknowledged in the article. Writing satire means treading a fine line between obscurity and absurdity. Two

examples of this from recent years are 'Sister Plume' in *Nursing Times* (apparently a traditionalist old battleaxe dispensing advice to junior nurses) and 'Sister Susie' in *Nursing Standard* (a trendy young ward leader with endless enthusiasm for management fads and jargon).

It is worth experimenting, as you may need to use different approaches for different topics and for different journals over the years. Keeping to one approach may help you develop your style more quickly, but it limits the market for your work, partly because it limits the number of journals to which you can submit, and partly because editors are always looking for something new, and may quickly lose interest in a series of similar pieces.

KNOWING THE JOURNAL

If you know which approach you are taking, or which one you want to try out, then you need to find a journal which takes that type of article. You will know from your background reading which publications include humorous perspective pieces, and which run satirical columns or spoof quizzes. In addition to this research, it is worth remembering that:

- some journals will use humorous pieces for special occasions, even if they don't normally publish this type of article. Christmas, or significant anniversaries, are such examples of occasions (I had a couple of humorous articles published around the time of the 50th anniversary of the National Health Service – mainly, I suspect, because people were running out of nurses/patients/doctors who admitted to being in the NHS on its first day)
- sometimes editors can be persuaded to take something in a form they have not used before, so previous types of article need not be a rigid guide to future submissions.

If you have decided on your topic and your angle, but not on the approach, then you could look through the journals to see what kind of articles they have printed before, and then match your approach to this. If, for example, the *Journal of Clinical Idiocy* has included some spoof examination papers in the past, you might decide to write your piece on the differences between nursing in hospital and in the community in the style of a multiple-choice paper:

1. *Why do nurses move from acute to community nursing?*
    (a) to get closer to patients
    (b) to get further away from managers
    (c) to get better hours
    (d) to get better cars.

On the other hand, if you found a publication that had a regular 'readers' experiences' page, you might write it in narrative form:

> *Leaving the hospital for two weeks' experience in the community was like being a third-class passenger on the Titanic: everyone was terrified, no one seemed to know where to go, and there were definitely not enough life-boats.*

If you spotted an opportunity for more 'way out', satirical pieces you might take up the 'alien' angle:

> *Mission Control, this is Trust Voyager: we are about to disembark. Can you confirm all life support systems are A-okay?*
> *Mission Control to Trust Voyager, confirm blue felt hats and bicycles are suitable for planet's atmosphere. You are okay to go.*
> *Control, we are seeing some... ah, alternative support systems down here. We see transportation with four, repeat, zero four, wheels.*

APPROACHING THE EDITOR

This is an area where the steps involved in serious and humorous writing diverge. For serious articles, it is always worth talking to the editor before writing the article. They will be able to tell you whether they are interested in the topic, whether they have already commissioned articles on the subject, what they would like covered in any article you write, and what content, angle and length they require. It is much more difficult to discuss humorous pieces in detail with an editor. After all, what can you say? ('I'm going to write this hilariously witty piece on professional self-regulation...'.)

If you have definitely identified a journal which publishes the type of humorous article you want to write, then it is probably as well to write it and send it in, rather than discuss it with the editor first. However, you should write a slightly more detailed letter than usual to accompany the piece, explaining:

- why you think the topic will be of interest to the journal's readers
- why a humorous approach is appropriate (e.g. a new perspective on an old topic, or making a dull topic more interesting). This helps the editor to justify the decision to include the article, if challenged.

If you are not sure whether the journal that you are targeting will take your type of article, then you may need to ring the editor. However, instead of discussing your idea in the kind of detail you would normally expect for a clinical article, just check the general approach. For example, would they be interested in a light-hearted piece about video cameras in the labour suite?

Be prepared for more rejections with humorous articles than with serious clinical articles. Humour is risky for the journal as well as for the writer, and editors vary in their willingness to take that risk, as well as in their own brand of humour.

☛ **Rejection by an editor does not mean that the piece is not a good article, or that it is not funny. It may well find a market elsewhere.**

WRITING THE PIECE

Successful humorous writing probably cannot be learned from scratch, but it can be practised and polished. Some basic dos and don'ts are listed below.

DO:

- read as much humorous writing as you can find
- develop your style and 'voice' by writing several pieces together
- try to develop a number of different styles or approaches
- be prepared to discard some earlier attempts
- be as original as possible in topics and style, and in your voice
- match the topic to the journal you are targeting as closely as possible.

☛ **It is vital to avoid looking like a humorist in search of an outlet!**

DON'T:

- try too hard (e.g. by including jokes in your piece)
- mirror another writer's style or approach exactly
- flog a format (editors will start looking for something more original)
- expect to be published every time
- be gratuitously offensive to provoke laughs.

☛ **It would be impossible to write humorous material without ever offending anyone, but it is important to avoid the obvious traps, such as making humour out of death, disfigurement or disability.**

WORDS OF WARNING

Some people consider that there is no place for humorous writing in professional journals, and they will write to you and/or the journal to object. You cannot afford to be too sensitive to this if you want to continue to write in this vein.

Similarly, there will be people who will accept this kind of writing, but will take issue over your choice of topic. There is no such thing as 'fair game'! The defence

'But it's funny' cuts no ice with the defenders of whichever sacred institution you have targeted. For example, the UKCC, frilly hats for nurses, Project 2000 and politically correct health promotion campaigns all have their champions and, in my experience, readers are far more likely to write to authors about humorous pieces than about clinical articles.

You do not have the same excuses. You can hardly claim that you are writing silly satirical pieces for your professional development, or because you need a record of publications for the academic post on which you have set your heart. The best defence is that you aimed to amuse and entertain, and perhaps to encourage readers to take a fresh perspective on the topic. You did not intend to offend, but you are grateful that they have drawn their concerns to your attention. You should then file or throw away their letter, and get on with your next piece.

WORDS OF ENCOURAGEMENT

There are also many nice people in the world who will write you letters or rush up to you at conferences and say 'I love your pieces in the journal, they're brilliant, they always make me laugh'. This makes all the risks of humorous writing worthwhile. On no account should any such letters be thrown away, but rather they should be filed, or preferably framed, close to your desk to provide you with encouragement.

SUMMARY

Humorous writing needs to be practised and refined, and carefully targeted at an appropriate journal, in order to be successful. A variety of approaches can be used, and it is useful to develop more than one style, and to write for a range of different publications. The best preparation (and continuing education) in humorous writing is reading other people's work. It is worth being prepared to receive some criticism as well as some credit for this kind of writing.

CHAPTER ELEVEN

How to turn your dissertation into an article

This chapter looks at how you can use some of the hard work and agony that went into writing your dissertation to produce an article for publication in a professional journal. Fortunately, many of the same principles apply equally to turning any other piece of existing writing into an article. Project reports, essays and assignments for courses can all be reincarnated as publishable (and profitable) articles. There is only one golden rule for these transformations:

☞ **Do not send a dissertation (or any other existing piece of writing) unaltered to a journal for publication.**

There are four simple reasons for this rule.

- It will not be suitable for a journal article in its present form.
- The editor and/or reviewers will always recognise it for what it really is.
- You will lose credibility with the editor for appearing to think that it will be suitable for publication.
- If you are lucky, and the editor is particularly kind and patient, you will be asked to revise it for publication, so you will have to do the work in any case.

It is entirely understandable that, after all the work you have put in to prepare a dissertation or assignment for its original purpose, you are not inclined to start again with the same material to write a new piece. Fortunately, you are not really starting again, just adapting, reworking or revising – call it anything but 'starting again' if it helps!

WHY PUBLISH IT ANYWAY?

If the dissertation has fulfilled its original purpose, why bother to produce an article from it at all? The best reason in my opinion is to gain some more credit for the work you have put in. With a piece of work and writing of such magnitude, it seems a terrible waste for it to be read only by you, your supervisor and the external examiner. Of course, there are other and better reasons for publishing the work:

- to build up your professional reputation and so your career opportunities
- as a further educational exercise for you
- to contribute to the education of others in the profession.

However, as explained above, a dissertation, project report or assignment cannot be published as it stands. The main reason for this is that the piece was written to fulfil a different purpose, and whatever it was, it is most unlikely to match the reasons why articles are published in journals (*see* Box 11.1).

Box 11.1:   Comparison of the purposes of an article and of a dissertation

Purposes of dissertation	Purposes of article
To demonstrate learning about the research process	To inform or educate journal readers
To describe a piece of empirical research	To disseminate findings or implications of research to relevant others
To demonstrate competence in writing up research	To contribute to the professional development of the author

---

There are other practical barriers to the publication of unaltered reports, dissertations or assignments.

- They are probably of the wrong length. A dissertation may be anything from 15 000 to 30 000 words in length, and a journal article is more likely to contain 5000 words maximum. On the other hand, a project report may have 500 words, while a journal would require at least 1000 words.
- The phraseology will be wrong. The 'academic' style often adopted for dissertations, and the technical research language used, would not be suitable for many professional publications. Similarly, the detailed local service and personnel information included in a project report would not be appropriate in a journal article about the project.

- The emphasis will be different. A dissertation is intended to demonstrate the student's understanding of the subject, and their learning on the course, as well as their use of research methodology, practice and interpretation. Therefore there is usually a detailed explanation of the process of the research, including the rationale for discarding other methodologies, and a comprehensive review of previous research and literature on the subject. A journal article, by contrast, will need to emphasise the implications for clinical practice, or for the application of the research evidence to healthcare practice.

While this may all sound very obvious, I have reviewed many 'articles' which have been sent to professional journals for publication, and which are clearly other pieces of work that are not even thinly disguised. Some even contain phrases such as 'This report for the Trust Board will show how...' or 'In this assignment, I will discuss...'

It is obvious what has happened in such cases. Someone has said to the writer, 'That's really good, you should publish it', and the writer has thought, 'Mm, I'll give it a try, send it on the rounds'. Sadly, the usual scenario is that the article is then rejected, or recommended for revision by the author, and the writer sends it unaltered to a second journal. The same thing happens again, and the writer gives up, thinking 'Oh well, I did try – so much for disseminating professional knowledge'.

However, there is an alternative. By discussing the idea with an editor, and reworking the piece to suit a specifically targeted journal, the writer can be published, paid (sometimes) and receiving all the credit they deserve in the same time that it would take to receive the two rejection letters!

MATERIAL TO SAVE

Turning a dissertation or report into an article does not mean throwing out everything you have written already and starting again. Much of the content of the original piece can be reused, often exactly as it stands, in the article. For example, from a dissertation describing a piece of research, the 'bones' which can be extracted and reused include:

- the background reading and references
- the description of and rationale for the methodology used
- the results tables, charts or text
- the discussion
- the conclusions.

Of course, some of the content of these sections will have to be omitted, if only for reasons of length. However, it is much easier to start with too much material and then to extract the key points than to start from scratch.

☞ **Although some sentences or paragraphs can be transferred unchanged to the article, be ruthless about this. Do not include a section just because you were really pleased with the way it read, if it isn't essential to the new, leaner piece!**

From a project report, you can expect to salvage:

- the description of the situation which led to the setting up of the project
- the description of the way in which the project was set up
- the experiences of the professionals and clients involved
- the outcomes for clients
- lessons learned for implementation elsewhere (if included).

In fact, the only parts of a project report which are not useful in a journal article are the details of costing and finance arrangements, and of staffing.

FIRST STEPS

As with any article, when turning a dissertation into an article it is essential to be clear about:

- the topic of the piece
- the target readership
- its purpose.

Defining the topic is not quite as simple as it sounds, because it is not necessarily the same as the topic of your dissertation. You could, of course, aim to produce an article which simply summarised your dissertation. If the dissertation described a survey of intensive-care nurses' emotional attachment to their patients, the article could take the results of the survey as its topic. However, that is not the only option. The dissertation encapsulates a whole range of different pieces of work which took place around the survey, and any of these could form the topic for the article. For example, the article could focus on the literature search. Perhaps it showed that there is very little research into this area, or that the results of existing research are contradictory. An article on this topic could be written for a specialist journal targeting intensive-care-unit nurses, to stimulate discussion and debate.

Alternatively, the article could focus on the experience of conducting the survey itself. It could be aimed at all nurses, via one of the weekly journals, and intended simply to entertain with tales of nurses' aversion to researchers, and the excuses they provide for non-cooperation.

A third option would be to focus specifically on the methodology used, discussing the pros and cons and the ethics of using self-completion surveys rather than interview techniques, when the population surveyed are professionals at work.

There are invariably many options for article topics arising from any one piece of work (*see* Box 11.2). Rather than choosing between them and writing just one piece, it is of course possible to write several different articles on different topics from one dissertation. This is sometimes known as 'salami publishing' – slicing up the dissertation into different pieces.

Box 11.2: Options for article topics from leg ulcer research

Options for articles based on research into the assessment skills of district nurses caring for patients with leg ulcers could include:

- an opinion piece about nurses and record-keeping
- a review of the literature on standardised assessment tools for leg ulcers
- an educational article on the national standard for holistic assessment of patients with leg ulcers
- a descriptive article about the training received by district nurses prior to assessing leg ulcers
- a humorous piece about the experience of working with the Trust audit department.

The questions of who the article is written for, and why, also have to be addressed – as for any other article.

☞ **Just because the article comes from a dissertation, it does not have to be aimed at an academic audience via the most forbidding journal on the library shelves.**

However, if academic credit is what you are looking for, then you will need to target an audience of academics, researchers and educationalists. If you don't already read an appropriate journal, find one from the library shelves, or by discussing the matter with your research supervisor. Some of the journals which provided articles during your literature search might also be worth looking at for publication. If you are thinking of targeting a journal that you do not normally read, it is important to carry out the journal assessment described in Chapter 3. This includes finding out:

- who edits the journal
- who is on the journal staff
- the journal's aim or mission statement
- the targeted readership
- the types of articles they usually publish
- who writes for the journal
- what topics they have covered recently

- what topics, if any, they are 'trailing' for coverage in the near future
- how often the journal appears
- how long the delay is between acceptance of an article and its publication – it can be well over a year!

☞ **The date on which an article was accepted often appears at the bottom of the first page of the article in research journals.**

It is not necessary to target an academic or research journal with an article arising from a dissertation. The weekly nursing magazines, clinical and specialist journals all publish articles describing research, with an emphasis on the implications of the findings for clinical practice. It may be less daunting to produce an article for these journals than for a research journal, particularly for a less experienced writer. This does not mean that the publication is less valuable to the profession, even if the purists would regard it as less valuable to the aspiring academic. Almost all of these publications are now 'peer reviewed' – that is, they send articles out to one or more expert referees before deciding whether to accept them. The process is not as rigorous as that undertaken by an international research journal, but neither is it the case that any research project will be accepted for publication in the journal regardless of its merit.

☞ **Plenty of research is undertaken, but very little is routinely incorporated into practice. Publishing in the journals that are read by practising nurses can be your contribution to redressing this imbalance!**

Thus if your target audience consists of general nurses, or people working in a particular speciality, and your purpose is to inform, educate, spread good practice or stimulate discussion, the general or specialist clinical journals might well be the right place to target. Whether you choose a general or specialist journal will also depend on the nature of the research or project you are reporting. If the research looked at the patient assessment skills of district nurses working with leg ulcers, and the topic of the article is the research findings, a specialist community nursing or wound care journal will provide the most appropriate readership. However, if the topic of the article is the criterion-based audit of medical records, which was the methodology for the research, then it could be targeted at a general nursing audience, for application to any clinical topic – or to an even wider audience.

WIDENING THE NET

This last example highlights another of the options available to a dissertation that has been turned into an article: it need not be limited to the writer's professional journals. Many aspects of the work undertaken for the research project will have multidisciplinary implications or interest. For example, a specialist nurse's investigation into self-medication for back pain could be of interest to physiotherapists as well as community nurses – and the use of significant event analysis as an audit tool to assess palliative care is relevant to a whole range of professions. Therefore it is worth investigating unfamiliar journals in other fields when deciding how to target the article. In addition to unidisciplinary publications, there are multidisciplinary journals which welcome articles from a wide range of health professionals – for example, the *Journal of Clinical Excellence* and *Primary Health Care Research and Development* (*see* Box 11.3).

Box 11.3:   Two examples of multidisciplinary journals

Primary Health Care Research and Development

Aimed at a wide range of practitioners in primary health care
A forum for researchers and practitioners to debate issues and exchange information
International and interdisciplinary
Welcomes papers which disseminate evidence, information and practice examples of research and developmental activities

Journal of Clinical Excellence

Designed to influence and challenge clinicians and managers responding to the work of the National Institute for Clinical Excellence
Welcomes contributions on clinical governance, national service frameworks, clinical indicators, implementing change, clinical effectiveness and audit, and professional development

---

TALKING TO THE EDITOR

Although there is generally a set format for research report articles (*see* Box 11.4), and individual journals give explicit instructions about word length, number of tables, and so on, it is still worth talking to the editor about this type of article. They can tell you whether they are interested in the topic, and whether they already have a similar article in preparation. By letting them know that you are writing the article, you also give them an opportunity to fit it in with a special themed edition, if they have one (e.g. on elderly care or community nursing). If they want to do this, it will affect the deadline that they suggest.

If you are not planning a traditional research report, it is even more important that you talk to the editor to establish:

● their interest in the topic

- their view of the approach you are planning
- how your article might fit with planned articles, themes and special editions
- the word length and deadline that are required by the journal.

Box 11.4:   The usual headings for a research report

- Introduction
- Literature review
- Aims of study
- Method
- Results/findings
- Analysis/discussion
- Summary/conclusion

Most journals also ask for an abstract (a brief summary of all of the sections, which appears at the beginning of the printed article) and the identification of up to six 'key words' (which will be used for indexing the article in databases).

☞ **Remember, if the editor accepts the idea and your approach to it, you are at least three-quarters of the way to publication!**

PLANNING THE ARTICLE

The difference between planning an article from your dissertation and planning any other article from scratch is that you have already written much of the content. Part of your planning is to divide up the content and background you have between the sections of the article. You therefore need to decide on the sections first, remembering all the time that the purpose of the article is different to the original purpose of the dissertation.

For example, consider an article being planned from a dissertation by a dietitian.

Dissertation author: a dietitian.
Dissertation topic: research undertaken for an MSc.
Research topic: the nutritional value of the diet of nursery-age children.
Methodology: the parents of the class population of 30 nursery children from an affluent semi-rural area completed detailed food diaries for their children for 1 month. These were analysed by the dietitian, and compared to national recommendations regarding child nutrition.
Findings: 30% of the children received less than the recommended daily amount of iron, vitamin A (and many other alarming findings). Parents cited health

professionals, especially health visitors, as their main source of advice about child nutrition.

Conclusion: research is needed to find out why affluent parents do not provide their children with nutritionally adequate diets (and to answer other questions); health professionals working with young families need to check parents' understanding of nutrition.

The dietitian decides to make the topic of her article the nutritional information given to parents by health visitors. It is aimed at a readership of health visitors, via *Community Practitioner*, the journal of the Community Practitioners' and Health Visitors' Association, and is intended to give them information to consolidate their practice.

The section headings for this article could be as follows:

Introduction
Background to child nutrition
Evidence for the problem
Parents and nutritional information
The health visitor's role
Conclusion.

Some of the content of the original dissertation could then be divided among these sections. However, there will also need to be some new material, particularly in the introduction, which describes the aim of the article. These elements of the planning are shown in Box 11.5.

Clearly, much of the original material from the dissertation cannot appear in this article. The detailed literature review of studies of nutrition in young children cannot be reproduced in the short article, nor can the exhaustive explanation of the methods of qualitative analysis of the diaries. This information must be excluded from this article, although it could of course form the main topic of two more articles.

WRITING THE ARTICLE

Again, the principle here is to be ruthless with the dissertation material. Use sentences or even whole paragraphs from the dissertation if they are necessary and appropriately worded. However, you should not use them just because they have a nice turn of phrase or they sound wonderfully academic and intelligent.

☞ **With this type of article it is a good idea to ask someone else to read it through and see if it appears logical and complete, as you will be too familiar with the material to detect any gaps or inconsistencies.**

Box 11.5:   Turning dissertation content into article content

Section	Dissertation content	New content
Introduction	–	Aims of the article
Background to child nutrition	Some 'scene-setting' from the introduction Some references to relevant literature, guidelines, etc.	Involvement of health visitors with child nutrition
Evidence for the problem	Some references to relevant studies The new research findings Implications of findings	–
Parents and nutritional information	Some references to relevant studies	References to health visitor's role in advising parents on child nutrition
The health visitor's role	New research findings about parents' reliance on health visitors' advice	Discussion of potential impact of increased health visitor emphasis on child nutrition
Conclusion	Even some affluent parents lack information with which to provide an adequate diet for their young children	Health visitors can make a difference to the health of these children by reinforcing the dietary advice that is given to parents

---

SUMMARY

The key to publishing successfully from a dissertation is to accept that it will have to be rewritten to form an article. By identifying the topic, the target readership and the purpose of the piece, you can plan the section headings for the article in the usual way. The content of the dissertation or project report can then be inserted into the appropriate section or sections. Some of the content will have to be omitted because of the constraints of word length, and because this information is not necessary for the different purpose of the article, but it could form part of additional or subsequent articles.

CHAPTER TWELVE

How to get a book contract

Yes, you can! Many people whose instinctive reaction is 'I might write an article but I could never write a book' could in fact do just that. There are some provisos, of course, but generally speaking, if you can write an article you can write a book.

Writing a non-fiction book is in many ways like writing a whole series of articles in very quick succession. However, in some significant ways writing a book is quite different. The first major difference is the sometimes lengthy process to be undertaken in order to arrive at the point of even beginning to write the book! This process will be explained in this chapter, while the actual writing and the steps to publication will be dealt with in the next chapter.

How to begin?

There are two ways to begin the process of writing a book on a professional or clinical topic (the only type to be discussed in this chapter):

- waiting to be asked to contribute to someone else's book
- 'selling' your idea for a book to a publisher, so that they may offer you a contract to write it.

There are also two approaches which are generally non-starters:

- writing a book from scratch and then trying to sell it to a publisher – this is like cooking a seven-course banquet and then ringing your relatives in Australia and asking them to come over and eat it

☞ **Do not even contemplate writing your book without finding a publisher first!**

- writing a book when you have no previous experience of writing for publication – this is roughly equivalent to taking your first driving lesson on the M25 during a cloudburst in a Friday rush-hour. Not only is this difficult to do in itself, but you will have much more difficulty persuading a publisher to take on your book if you cannot demonstrate that you can write clearly, professionally and to a defined brief.

GETTING STARTED – THE EASY WAY

Probably the simplest way to start writing books is to wait to be invited to contribute a chapter to a multi-authored book. Such invitations are not uncommon. Editors (both individuals and commissioning editors working for publishers) are always looking for potential contributors who can combine clinical or organisational knowledge with the ability to write. One way in which they find them is by noting names on articles in the professional journals.

☞ **Publishing articles regularly is the best way to build up a reputation in a particular clinical area or in relation to a particular topic.**

It is easy to see from your own reading that certain names become associated with particular topics, and then turn up on the covers of books on the same topics. I have known this to happen to nurses who wrote regularly about travel medicine, immunisation, practice nursing and nursing homes, as well as to a practice manager who wrote about management and financial topics. Writing many articles on a subject, over a period of time and for a number of different journals, means that:

- you gather a large amount of background and reference material, which saves time when preparing future articles
- you keep up to date with developments in the field, and read the latest documents, so you are quick to spot potential topics for articles
- your name becomes associated with the topic in the minds of readers, editors and reviewers
- you develop the art of writing quickly and lucidly
- you become skilled at presentation of manuscripts, talking to editors, keeping to word length and meeting deadlines.

Therefore, while you are gaining all the necessary experience and skill to contemplate writing a book, commissioning editors are noting your name and your expertise and the scene is set for an approach. If this connection does not happen as fast as you would like it to, you could always take the initiative yourself (*see* Box 12.1 for ways to ensure that you are likely to be asked to contribute to a book sooner rather than later).

Box 12.1:   Inviting invitations to write a chapter

If you want to write a chapter for a book, and no one has asked you to yet, you could try:

- asking relevant tutors at the local Department of Nursing whether they know of anyone planning a book on your subject
- contacting commissioning editors at the types of publishers that are likely to produce books on the subject, to ask whether they know of an editor looking for contributors
- talking to the editors of appropriate specialist journals, for the same reason
- advertising for 'collaborators' in the nursing press.

THE OFFER

You will probably be contacted by letter (forwarded from one of the journals you write for regularly) or by telephone at your place of work, if your contact details have appeared at the end of one of your articles. The initial approach may be from the commissioning editor of a publishing company interested in the proposed book, or from an individual who is planning to edit a multi-authored book, and who has either already talked or intends to talk to the commissioning editor. The editor's letter or telephone call will describe the proposed book, and the chapter or section they would like to commission from you. At this point, be polite and professional, but only express an interest in being involved in the project if:

- you know that you have time to produce the work
- you are sure that you can cover the topic they want in the way they want
- you are prepared to sign a contract to produce the agreed work
- you are prepared for the frustrations and compromises inherent in collaboration.

☞ Ask to see a copy of the full proposal for the book, so that you know who else is writing, what else is covered in the book, the target readership, the date for completion, and so on. All of these factors will affect the way in which you write your contribution, and even whether you want to be involved at all!

For example, as a well-known writer on professional issues affecting nursing homes, you might be asked to contribute a chapter about nursing in the independent sector. If the book to which you are contributing is a handbook about alternative career paths for newly qualified nurses, you might be pleased to contribute. However, if it is about accountability and professional misconduct, with the emphasis on misconduct in the private sector, you might not be so keen.

If you have expressed an interest in writing the chapter, you should receive a letter setting out the terms of the commission. These will include:

- the content of your chapter or section
- the word length required
- the deadline for delivery
- the way in which you will be paid (*see* Box 12.2)
- the amount you will be paid.

Usually there will be an agreement for you to sign to indicate your acceptance of these terms. You may well want to discuss the commission in detail with the editor before making a decision. It is important that you are absolutely clear about what is required, that you can provide it, and that you have the time to meet the deadline indicated.

Box 12.2:   Royalties versus commission

These are the two principal ways in which you are likely to be paid for your writing

Royalties

- are a percentage of the net sales receipts received by the publisher from the sale of your book
- are often set at around 10–12.5%
- are paid twice a year
- are entirely dependent on the 'success' of the book, as measured by the volume of sales

Commission

- is a once-only payment
- is often around £100 per chapter
- is paid after publication, as for a journal article
- is unrelated to subsequent sales of the book

☞ **Don't sign the form unless you can meet the terms to which you are agreeing!**

WRITING THE CHAPTER

Writing the chapter or section is much the same as writing an article. You need to be clear about the topic, the target readership, and the purpose of the chapter. The difference is that all of these things are decided not by you alone, but by you and the editor together. You may well have to compromise frequently, and sometimes significantly, during this process.

👉 **Remember, it may be your chapter, but it's their book!**

This is one reason why it is so important to talk to the editor, asking questions and defining exactly what is required, before you sign an agreement to write the chapter. If, for example, the editor has in mind a practical handbook on wound dressing, aimed at practising nurses, and you usually write theoretical and academic articles based on your research into the psychology of altered body image, there are quite likely to be problems. Of course, editors would usually choose their contributors more appropriately, but misunderstandings do occur. Setting up an agreement is a two-way process, and the writer shares the responsibility for ensuring that they are a good match with the requirements of the book proposal.

However, assuming that you are the right person to write the chapter, and that the topic is one you can comfortably cover in the required word length and to the deadline specified, what could possibly go wrong? Unsurprisingly, there are several potential sources of frustration involved in contributing to someone else's book.

- The editor may ask for changes to style or approach in order to be consistent with other chapters.
- You may not see any of the other chapters until the book is published.
- You may not like the other chapters, with which yours will be associated, when you do see them.
- You may receive little information about the progress of the project.
- Other contributors may fail to submit their chapters on time, and so delay the whole process.
- The process may be delayed for technical reasons, and you may feel that your chapter has lost its topicality, or appears out of date, because of this.

You may feel that having your name on a chapter in a book is sufficient compensation for facing these difficulties. If not, perhaps you will decide to take more control of the process in future by developing that idea you had for writing your own book...

GETTING STARTED – THE HARDER WAY

If no one asks you to contribute to their book, or you have had enough of writing for other people and decide to write a book of your own, then the first thing you need to do is sell your idea to a publisher. Remember:

👉 **Do not write a book before you have found a publisher for it!**

In order to obtain a contract or agreement with a publisher, you will have to convince the commissioning editor that:

- there is a market for your book – that is, lots of people who will want to buy it
- your book contains something different to all the other books currently in print on the same subject
- you have the clinical, technical or other relevant expertise to write on the subject
- you can write
- you will be able to deliver the agreed number of words, in the agreed format, to an agreed deadline.

The formal way to do this is to prepare a 'book proposal' for the publishers. However, this is only one of several steps on the way to obtaining a contract (*see* Box 12.3).

Box 12.3:   Essential preparatory steps involved in obtaining a contract to write a book

- Plan the topic and scope of the book.
- Investigate the possible publishers for your type of book.
- Discuss your idea with a commissioning editor from the chosen publishers.
- Prepare a detailed proposal for the book, for consideration by the commissioning editor, editorial board and reviewers.

PLANNING THE TOPIC

Just as with identifying a topic for an article, a broad heading such as 'asthma', 'nurse prescribing' or 'health promotion' is no help at all. It is essential to be clear exactly what aspect of the topic is to be covered in the book. This in turn depends on both the intended readership and the purpose of the book. For example, on the topic of nurse prescribing, the proposed publication could be:

- a handbook for potential nurse prescribers, to refer to in daily practice
- a textbook to support their initial training, including exercises and case studies
- a commentary on the legal and ethical aspects of prescribing, aimed at all clinicians who have (or may acquire) prescribing rights
- a collection of different perspectives on the development of nurse prescribing, from multidisciplinary contributors.

Each of these books would take a different approach to the topic of nurse prescribing, and would contain different information presented in a different format.

In pinning down the topic and approach, you need to be able to answer three key questions.

- What exactly is it about?
- Who is it aimed at?
- What is it intended to do?

As an example, the answers to these questions for this book are shown in Box 12.4.

Box 12.4:   The key questions and answers involved in planning this book

Question: What exactly is it about?
Answer: How to write articles or books for publication in the professional nursing and healthcare press.
Question: Who is it aimed at?
Answer: Nurses, therapists and midwives who have either not written for publication at all, or who have had a few articles published and want to write regularly.
Question: What is it intended to do?
Answer: Help the reader to prepare a publishable manuscript and/or move on to producing a book.

KNOWING THE PUBLISHERS

Once you have a clear idea what you want to write about, for whom and why, then you can set out to find an appropriate publisher to approach. Since it is a clinical or professional-type book, the range of publishers to be considered is immediately reduced to those specialising in these fields. There is no point approaching Mills and Boon or Penguin Classics!

To find out which publishers might be suitable, you could look through a list of all book publishers in the UK, such as that contained in the *Writers' and Artists' Yearbook*, published annually by A & C Black. The publishers' entries include the types of books they publish, so it is possible to draw up a short list of those which publish nursing or healthcare textbooks. Alternatively, you can do your own research by looking at existing books. You can find them by:

- looking in the local nursing library
- browsing in bookshops
- borrowing publishers' catalogues from librarians

- visiting publishers' exhibition stands at conferences
- visiting publishers' web sites on the Internet
- reading the book reviews and checking mail-order book-lists in the professional journals that you read
- checking your own and friends' bookshelves at home
- visiting the hospital or health centre 'resource centre' or library.

When searching the library or bookshop shelves, do not limit yourself to the section on the exact topic you are thinking of writing about. Look more generally at a wide range of nursing or healthcare textbooks, to find out:

- the names of the publishers
- what kinds of book each publisher produces (edited, multi-authored books, or books by single or dual authors; standard textbooks or distance-learning materials)
- what approach their books take (thick academic-looking texts, or shorter, more accessible 'handbooks' or 'workbooks')
- the visual appearance of their books (sober, plain covers, or brightly coloured binding; hardback or softback; large A4-size workbooks or pocket-size guides).

☞ **While you are looking at the different publishers' books, check the list of 'other publications' on the back cover, or in the front pages, to check that they have not already published something similar to your idea.**

Doing this kind of preliminary research will quickly identify a handful of companies that publish the type of book you have in mind – a simple step, but highly recommended (*see* Box 12.5 for several ways *not* to choose a publisher).

Box 12.5:   How not to choose a publisher

There are several tempting but inadvisable ways to choose a publisher. They usually end in rejection, embarrassment, wasted time or, quite frequently, all three. You are therefore advised not to:

- choose any publisher from a list at random
- go for the most prestigious and well-known name
- start at the letter 'A' and work through every publisher in alphabetical order
- target a publisher who has never produced a book like yours before.

Choosing which one of the short-listed publishers to approach first will then be a matter of personal preference (perhaps one in the same part of the country or, if you know anyone who has already published a book, one recommended to you).

APPROACHING THE PUBLISHERS

It is possible to debate endlessly the relative merits of sending a letter of enquiry to a publisher, or telephoning instead. A workable compromise is to telephone to ask for the name of the commissioning editor in the relevant area (e.g. nursing, medicine, education, or whatever covers your topic). If they are available, you could then speak to them about your idea; if not, you can write to them by name.

Sooner or later you are likely to have a telephone conversation with the commissioning editor. This is an opportunity to sell your idea, the market for it, and yourself as the writer, much as you would sell an article idea to a journal editor.

☛ **Have these points clear in your mind, and preferably on paper, before you telephone the publisher, as you might find yourself having to make an immediate sales pitch to a commissioning editor.**

The difference between selling an idea for an article and one for a book is that, with a book, there is a 'next stage', namely the book proposal. Provided that you have chosen an appropriate publisher in the first place, and have been at least mildly convincing to the commissioning editor, you will probably be invited to write a proposal for your book. The editor will send you some guidelines on the content of the proposal, and will suggest a date for you to submit it.

☛ **Naturally, as this is your first deadline from your potential publisher, you must make sure that you meet it!**

The editor will also probably invite you to contact him or her to discuss the proposal as you write it, if you wish. This is a genuine offer, and often a very useful one for both sides, as it is in everyone's best interests to have a complete, appropriately structured and precisely targeted proposal at the time of first submission.

THE PROPOSAL

The purpose of any book proposal is to make the publisher want to commission and publish the book. It is quite simply a sales tool for you – a place for confidence, accurate detail, convincing information and professional presentation.

The format of the proposal is set by the guidelines issued by the publisher. The information usually required in a proposal is shown in Box 12.6. So how should you set about filling in the sections?

Box 12.6:   Content of a typical book proposal

The publisher will send an outline for a proposal in the format that they want.
The proposal usually contains the following information:

- background/introduction
- aims and scope of the book
- style and approach
- target market
- competing/complementary texts
- list of chapters/content of chapters
- length
- the qualifications and experience of the author(s) or contributor(s).

BACKGROUND/OUTLINE

This is an opportunity to say in a few sentences something about the context of the
book – the changes, new developments, different ideas or recent events which have
convinced you of the need for a new book on the topic. It is also worth describing the
proposed book in a succinct sentence or two at this early stage in the proposal, to
give the editor a clear idea of what they are being asked to look at. For example:

- 'a practical handbook on caring for people in their own homes, for student nurses
  doing community placements'
- 'a textbook on travel medicine and immunisation, for GPs and practice nurses'
- 'a directory of complementary therapies in palliative care, for doctors, nurses and
  therapists working with people with terminal illness'
- 'a practical guide to managing a nursing home, for nurse managers in the
  independent sector'.

THE MARKET

The proposal needs to identify the specific target market for the book. The more
precisely the target market is defined, the easier it is for the publisher's marketing
department to sell it, and therefore recoup the cost to the publisher of producing it. A
target market of 'nurses' or 'therapists' is likely to be much too vague to be useful.
Try to focus on the subgroup which is most likely to buy the book (e.g. nurses in a
particular speciality or on a particular course; a specific type of therapist, working
with specific client groups, or at a certain stage of their careers).

The proposal guidelines from the publisher will often ask for an estimate of the numbers in the target market, and with a little research it is usually possible to find out an approximate figure. For example, the number of training places per year on particular courses, or the number of certain specialist nurses can be obtained from various professional bodies or associations.

You may also be asked to provide information about 'secondary markets' – that is, people other than those specifically targeted who may want to buy the book. Resist the temptation to suggest that there are huge secondary markets for your book. The publisher is not likely to be able to spend time and money marketing to many different groups in a variety of different ways (and it usually looks like grasping at straws).

☞ **Numbers are not everything – better to have a clearly defined group, many of whom can be persuaded to buy the book, than a huge but ill-defined field which is impossible to target.**

You may also be asked if there is an international readership for your subject. Be realistic about this – it will depend on how transferable your subject is to different healthcare systems and cultures. A clinical topic (e.g. prevention of strokes) will 'travel' better than one specific to the English part of the National Health Service (e.g. setting up primary care groups).

TIMING

If there is any reason to support the publication of a book on your topic at the time when you are proposing to write it, it is worth including in the proposal. Examples might include:

- the advent of a new issue in health care (current examples are clinical governance or nurse prescribing)
- a new course (as the specialist practitioner degree programmes were in the mid-1990s)
- the implementation of new technologies (drugs, treatments or services)
- renewed interest in the topic (such as ethics, genetics or health screening).

Linking your book to something new is a powerful argument for publication, particularly for a perennial topic. Why should a publisher produce yet another textbook on public health, unless it is because the Government health programme is focusing more and more on collective action for health? A handbook on audit methodologies might seem entirely superfluous, unless it is linked to the new statutory duty for clinical governance, which requires participation in audit.

☞ **Remember that it can take around a year from delivery of a manuscript to publi-**

cation of a book, and perhaps a year before that to write it! Topicality is, by definition, ephemeral, so be sure that the 'new' thing to which you are linking your book will last at least until it is published!

Some publishers can produce books on a topical subject much more quickly. If you can write it quickly (say in 6 months) they may produce the book in another 4–5 months. This works best for topics which have a well-defined target audience and a clear 'window of opportunity' during which they can be marketed to the target readership.

One example is the setting up of primary care groups (PCGs) in April 1999. An impressive number of books were published in the months immediately before and after this date, specifically targeting the GPs, nurses and managers who were starting out in these new organisations. The primary target market was clearly defined and quantifiable (number of PCGs × 13 members of each PCG Board, plus number of health authorities × (say) 10 managers each, etc.). The secondary market consisted of the rest of the GPs, community nurses and managers who would be directly affected by the PCGs. The majority of the books produced were very practical workbooks, handbooks and guides, rather than academic texts. The window of opportunity extended from 1998 (the preparatory year) to the end of 1999 (when the PCGs were in place).

If your idea is for something very topical with an externally defined time-scale, you should look for a publisher who is willing to produce these high-risk, fast-turnaround books.

COMPETING/COMPLEMENTARY TEXTS

In this section of the proposal you are expected to list the other books in the same field which might compete with your book for sales. Clearly, it is highly unlikely that you will be able to plan a book on a topic that no one has ever written about before. Therefore your aim is to show that your book either contains new information, perspectives or insights on the topic, or covers aspects which are not adequately covered for the target readership in existing books.

For example, many books have already been published on nursing in the community. It is by no means a new topic, and almost every aspect has been covered exhaustively by a range of books. However, I sold the idea to a publisher for my first book, on nursing in primary care, by stressing:

- the *new* emphasis on primary care nursing in pre-registration nursing courses
- the combination of primary care (GP practice) and community nursing perspectives, which was *different* to that of other competing texts
- the practical, 'dip-into' handbook format, which was *different* to the format of most competing texts.

If your topic is a relatively common one, the thought of listing and appraising all of the other books already on the market can be daunting. You can narrow down the list by restricting it to those publications which closely match the content of your proposed book. For example, rather than listing all of the current publications on 'mental health nursing', you could restrict it to 'nursing mentally ill adults in the community', if that is the subject of your book. You can further narrow the field by fixing a 'published since…' date. Books on the management of childhood asthma published in the last 10 years will be a far more manageable list than 'all books ever published on asthma in children'. You can narrow the field still further by concentrating on books which are aimed at the same target audience as yours. For example, books for nurses in clinical practice or nurses doing postgraduate degrees will exclude some of the textbooks on childhood asthma written for doctors taking advanced examinations.

☞ **Don't be too concerned about finding every single publication. This is not a comprehensive literature search – you are simply supporting your argument for your new book.**

Once you have established the parameters of your search, there are several easy ways to draw up the list of competing texts which you need to look at:

- browse the catalogue at your nursing library, using some relevant keywords to search among book titles
- consult the catalogues you may already have obtained when you were choosing a short list of publishers to target, to see what has been published in the last year or two
- look in the library or on the bookshelves at your place of work for existing textbooks relevant to your area of practice
- look at the book reviews and mail-order book-lists in some back issues of a relevant professional journal.

☞ **Don't give up if there seem to be a lot of existing books on the subject even after you have narrowed the search. Many of these will turn out not to be competitors.**

When I conducted the search for possible competitors to this book, I was dismayed to find shelves full of books on writing for nurses at the library. However, on closer examination it became apparent that the vast majority either related solely to American journals, or focused on writing dissertations and theses. Those that were about writing for the UK nursing press took a different viewpoint to the one I had in mind, so could be viewed as complementary rather than as competition.

Once you have a list of books which could be regarded as competitors to your own, you need to review them briefly to demonstrate why they do not render your book unnecessary. Some of the reasons you might find are listed in Box 12.7.

Box 12.7:   Why competing texts might not render a new book unnecessary

Very few books have the advantage of being launched into virgin territory. However, the fact that books on the same subject exist need not rule out the need for another. The 'competitors' may be:

- aimed at a different market
- out of date (even within a year or two!)
- about a different country/healthcare system
- taking a different approach
- written in a different style
- written at a different level.

👉 **It is only necessary to write a few sentences on each book, not a full book review!**

At the end of this section of the proposal, it is useful to put a summary sentence such as that shown in Box 12.8. This is part of the selling technique to convince the commissioning editor that you have already proved that they must publish your book!

Box 12.8:   Summary sentence about competing texts

Having dissected the competition, it is useful to summarise the gap in the market for the editor reading the proposal. For example:

Although there are many other texts on health promotion, there are none which are written by a practising midwife, and which focus specifically on practical interventions with mothers during pregnancy and in the perinatal period.

AIMS AND SCOPE/STYLE AND APPROACH

However it is titled, this is the section in which to describe the type of book you have in mind, the way it will look on the page, and the kind of writing it will contain. It is, of course, essential that these different elements are consistent both with each other and with the target readership. Some of the options that are available are listed in Box 12.9. Existing books will provide some guidance as to what is appropriate for different types of book and readership, although there are few unbreakable rules. Bear in mind, however, that it would be asking a lot of any publisher to risk producing the first 'pop-up' guide to neurological anatomy for doctors!

Box 12.9:   Options for style and approach

Books – even textbooks – are not all written in the same way. There are many different styles and approaches which are appropriate to different aims and different audiences. For example:

Style	Approach	Purpose
'Academic' text	Well referenced and discursive, uses models, tables and diagrams in moderation; written by respected experts/ academics	Background information, knowledge acquisition, for students on pre-registration and postgraduate courses, and for professional development
Handbook	More practically focused, uses diagrams, pictures, summary boxes, bullet points, etc., in addition to text; written by clinical experts/practising clinicians	Day-to-day guidance, 'dip into' reference, for practising clinicians or use in professional development activities/courses
Workbook	Very practical, uses all of the devices listed above, also features exercises, or 'things to do' as learning tools, sometimes has pages to use for notes, or to fill in; written by people with practical experience/ expertise	Training/education on a practical topic, for courses or professional development
Directory	Format is basically a list, with additional information about each entry; often produced by an organisation, but may be collated by an individual	Used to look up information on an *ad hoc* basis, usually by people who need a specific piece of information
Other	For example, ABC of... Factfinder on... Tips for... 100 ways to...	Quick references, can be aimed at students or clinicians in the field

LIST OF CONTENTS

This section demonstrates that you have given detailed thought to covering the subject of the book in an appropriate and comprehensive way. A book on complementary therapies for intensive-care-unit nurses sounds great, but if you can only cover a couple of therapies at a relatively superficial level, it may be difficult to convince the editor that it should be a book rather than an article.

☞ **If you are sharing the writing of a book with one or more other people, then the contributors' names should be given for each chapter.**

Each chapter title should be accompanied by a paragraph or list of bullet points indicating what is covered in the chapter. Taken together, the content of all of the chapters should match the aims and scope of the book as set out in the previous section. If you have described the book as a comprehensive text for child branch student nurses to prepare them for final examinations, but the chapters only cover half of the curriculum, then there is a serious mismatch which will have to be addressed.

☞ **Don't make general claims for the book which cannot be met in the detail of the chapters, or put detail in the chapters which is irrelevant to the aims.**

The list of chapters can be accompanied by a list of appendices which you plan to include. These often contain some of the most useful information in the book in an easily accessible form, and deserve a mention as part of the sales pitch.

LENGTH

How long is a piece of string? When I wrote my first book, I suggested in my proposal that it would be 15 000 words long. The editor kindly put me right, and we settled on 90 000. This book, by contrast, will be 35–40 000 words in length. So there is no standard single figure, or even range, which is necessarily 'right'.

☞ **Don't be afraid to ask for advice about word length from the commissioning editor as you are writing the proposal.**

ABOUT THE AUTHOR(S)

The section on the author(s) of the proposed book is the place to sell yourself (and your collaborators, if you have any) as the ideal person to write the book. This is not a CV, and you do not have to list every post you have ever held and everything you have ever written in chronological order. What is important here is to match your relevant experience to the skills that will be needed to write the book. Two categories of skills are relevant:

- your clinical/technical expertise – do you know enough about the topic of the book to be credible as the author?
- your writing skills – are you going to be able to deliver a well-written, publishable manuscript at the required word length and to the deadline?

To indicate your clinical/technical expertise, you will want to describe your relevant posts, experience, qualifications, and so on. Think of it like the blurb on the back of the book: 'So and so has worked in Accident and Emergency departments for the last 15 years, and currently manages the largest trauma centre in Scotland. He is also a part-time lecturer at Scotshire University, and has presented papers on emergency care at conferences in the UK and the US' (and presumably he is not writing a book about midwifery!).

Do not be put off if you don't have a lot of grand-sounding qualifications and job titles to offer. Your clinical experience, or your expertise in a different area, may be your selling point. The key point is that the information you offer about yourself matches the claims you are making for the book. If you are writing a practical handbook for practice nurses on dealing with minor injuries, you will need different experience and background to someone who is writing an academic text on the cultural differences between nursing and medicine, and the transfer of certain tasks between the professions.

☞ **Beware of implying that you are going to write the whole book from your personal experience. Make it clear that you have researched the area thoroughly (or will do so).**

To establish your writing abilities, it is very useful to be able to cite a number of different publications you have already produced. This is where your experience of writing articles for journals can pay dividends. It demonstrates to the editor that you are not just another wannabe author, one of the many people who are always talking about writing a book but are less likely to produce one than to discover a new solar system. Listing some of the articles you have written shows that:

- you can produce consistently coherent writing
- you have the time and discipline to write
- you can meet deadlines and write articles within pre-arranged word lengths
- you know how to correct proofs
- you understand something about the process of publication and the responsibilities of the writer.

Ideally you will be able to show that you have taken a similar approach in articles to that which you propose in the book – that is, if it is an educational book, you have written educational materials, and if it is an academic book, you have written research articles. However, any kind of published professional writing is a great boost to your claim to be ready and willing to write a book.

Do not despair if you have never written for publication before. Some people do start with a book. However, you should double-check with the rest of your life that you have the time, stamina, commitment and ability to do so.

WHAT HAPPENS NEXT?

Once your proposal is complete – and you might want to put a summary page at the back for the editor's convenience – it can be dispatched to the publisher for their consideration. Usually this will involve not only the commissioning editor, but consideration by an editorial board and a number of external reviewers as well. They will need to decide whether they think the book will be successful (i.e. marketable and profitable), and whether they are convinced by the proposal that you could write it. During these considerations you can expect to have some dialogue with the commissioning editor. They may send you copies of the reviewers' comments and suggestions, and discuss any elements of the proposal which are unclear or about which they are doubtful.

Although you do not have to accept every suggestion that is made about your proposal (and I have received some fairly unhelpful suggestions!), be prepared to be flexible about issues such as content, approach or timing. The editor, their editorial board and reviewers are experts in the publishing business, and their objectivity about your project can be very valuable. In addition, the process of writing and publication involves a lengthy working relationship between you and the editor, and too much intransigence at an early stage could scare them off!

☞ **It is not usually necessary to redraft the proposal and resubmit it to the publishers, but it is a good idea to alter your own copy when changes are agreed, because this will be the blueprint for your plan for the book.**

OUTCOME 1 – PASS

It may be that your proposal is turned down by the publishers after they have considered it. It is essential to remember that this does not mean that you cannot write a publishable book. There are a variety of reasons for rejection which need not be connected with the intrinsic merit of your proposal, or your perceived ability to write it. It is always worth discussing the reasons for rejection with the commissioning editor. They may be able to give you ideas about other publishers to approach, or aspects of your proposal which should be reworked before you approach another publisher.

OUTCOME 2 – THE CONTRACT

Once you have agreed the final details of the book, and if the editorial board decides to accept your proposal, the editor will send you a contract or 'memorandum of agreement'. The issues that are normally addressed in the contract are listed in Box 12.10.

Box 12.10:   Issues that are normally covered in the contract, or Memorandum of Agreement, between a publisher and an author or editor of a book

- The rights to be granted to the publisher
- The date and conditions for delivery of the manuscript
- The conditions for acceptance of the manuscript
- The publisher's responsibility to publish the book
- Copyright
- The scope of and procedure for corrections (both by the publisher and by the author)
- Royalties and commissions, and statements about sales
- Author's copies of the book
- Future revisions of the work
- Remainders and disposal of surplus stock
- Termination of the contract

☞ **As with any contract, read it carefully and do not sign it unless you are sure that you are prepared to be bound by all of its terms.**

Look particularly closely at the deadline, and be absolutely sure that you can meet it before you sign the contract. If it seems difficult to judge this, divide the number of chapters by the number of months before the deadline, and then ask yourself whether you are sure that you could write that number of chapters per month. This is when experience of writing articles can be very useful, as you will know how much time you can find for writing, and how many words you can produce over a given period.

SUMMARY

The steps involved in planning a book are similar to those in planning an article.

They include defining the topic of the book, getting to know the publishers in the field, and talking to the commissioning editor about your idea. An additional and very important step is the writing of a book proposal. Publishers have their own guidelines on preparing a proposal, which should be followed.

With a signed contract and a detailed proposal, you are ready to begin writing your book. Take a day off for serious celebration of this success, before moving on to the next chapter, which will guide you on how to write that book.

CHAPTER THIRTEEN

How to write that book

There was a period of time – say about 2 months – after I had signed my first book contract, in which I wandered about in a happy daze thinking 'I've got a book contract – I'm going to write a book – I'm going to be a proper author', and so on, day in and day out, during most conscious moments. What I should have been doing, of course, was writing the book.

☞ **The most difficult part of a big project such as writing a book is getting started. Try to get over that hurdle in the first week after signing the contract.**

In working out how long it would take you to write the book, during your negotiations with the commissioning editor, you will probably have broken down the task into manageable chunks – a chapter per month perhaps, or a section completed by Christmas. This timetable will be very useful to you during the writing process, so don't discard it as a mere theoretical exercise. Starting on time delays the moment when the planned timetable will inevitably slip, and the slippage time built into the plan will suddenly prove essential.

Making a start

Publishers will often send authors a set of guidelines on producing their manuscript. These will cover, among other things, their requirements for:

- page layout – margins, spacing, etc.
- text appearance – fonts, sizes, headings, spellings, etc.

- format for figures, tables, diagrams, references, etc.
- presentation of the manuscript – on both disk and on paper.

☞ **There is no place for whacky individuality here. The publishers want the manuscript in the format that suits them, so treat the instructions with reverent acquiescence, even if you do object to American spelling or Vancouver referencing.**

The first thing to do is to apply the formatting described to the first chapter document on the computer, so that you remember to follow the instructions throughout the months to come. (If you are not writing the book on a word processor yourself, but giving a manuscript to someone else to type, they will need to be given the guidelines, together with strict instructions to follow them religiously.)

The next step is to get something written as soon as possible. I used to find myself putting off starting a new chapter because 'between chapters' is such a tidy and satisfying place to be. Now I always stop working part of the way through a chapter, so that I can tell myself 'I'll just finish that chapter...'. Invariably I then get involved in the writing, finish one chapter and start the next before I stop working.

It is not necessary to start with the first chapter. Sometimes it is easier to start with another chapter, build some momentum, and then go back to write the first chapter. The detailed book proposal makes this a relatively simple thing to do, as there is no chance of forgetting what should be in each chapter, and in many ways each chapter can be treated as a separate entity. If you are not starting at Chapter 1, choose a chapter which:

- is relatively straightforward
- features a topic you are particularly enthusiastic about
- requires little extra research or information gathering.

An early 'success' in terms of a completed, well-written chapter which you enjoyed working on is a great incentive to continue the work.

APPROACHES TO WRITING

There are two main ways to approach writing a book.

- Make the logical progression of the book's content paramount, and write each chapter in order, rereading and revising from the beginning of the book.
- Treat the book as a series of separate pieces – revise each chapter as it is being written, and then set it aside and focus on another one.

The first approach has the advantage that, once you arrive at the end of the book, it is almost in its final form. The disadvantage is that the time spent going backwards and forwards over the text, perfecting each phrase as you go, can mean that the book soon falls behind schedule and there is far less time to spend on the last chapters than on the first few. It can also be difficult to read it objectively when you are constantly rereading it.

The second approach (treating each chapter like a separate article, and putting it aside once it is completed) means that you are likely to arrive at the end, with a set of completed chapters, somewhat sooner. However, the disadvantage of this approach is that some time has to be set aside at the end of the process for rereading the book as a whole, and making the inevitable additions and revisions to the chapters that were written in the early months.

No one way is better than another, but if you are an inexperienced writer and you try the first approach, watch your timetable carefully for potentially catastrophic slippage!

TIMING AND PACING

The importance of having a timetable alongside your book proposal cannot be overemphasised. Having a year to write a 50 000-word book might sound like plenty of time. However, if that breaks down into a chapter a month for 12 months, and in July you are away for a fortnight on holiday, and in February you have flu for 10 days, then keeping to the timetable becomes impossible.

The time to start tackling the problem of timing is at the proposal-writing stage. Suggest a deadline well after the time when you think you can actually deliver the book. If you then negotiate with the publishers because they are keen to publish earlier than your suggested deadline would allow, you must be insistent. If you bring forward the deadline, make sure that it is still further away than you think you need it to be.

When writing a book one thing is certain – it will always take longer than you think!

It can be helpful to mark some 'milestones' on your timetable, once the deadline is agreed (e.g. finishing the clinical section before Easter, or completing the first five chapters in 3 months). Achieving the milestones is a great psychological boost, and if you realise that the timetable is slipping because you reach the milestones late, then at least you are aware of the situation and can take remedial action.

With more time than you think you need, a prompt start after signing the contract, and a timetable with milestones on the wall to help you keep track of your progress, you are as well prepared as possible to deliver your manuscript on time.

If it looks remotely likely that you will not be able to meet the deadline, you must talk to your editor about it as soon as possible (see below).

Managing your life

However generous the deadline and however well planned and organised the book, it is still a certainty that the writing of it will disrupt your life. It is worth thinking, even before drafting a mental proposal for a book, what you will give up in order to write it. If you are working as well as writing a book, it is your evening and weekend activities (and probably some of your annual leave) that will have to be sacrificed. If you don't work outside the home, or if you work part-time, it is still unlikely that you have enough spare time now to be able to put in the hours necessary to produce a book without giving up something on which you currently spend time.

Writing my first book meant that I missed most of the season in which Macclesfield Town Football Club won promotion to Division Two. However, writing this one has meant that I have missed most of the season in which we slid inexorably back down into Division Three. Some sacrifices are just easier than others!

When people who have achieved amazing feats – running multinational companies whilst bringing up a family and baking their own bread, for example – are asked how they do it, they invariably say airily 'I suppose I'm just very organised' and, maddeningly simple as it is, that is probably the right answer. It certainly tops my list of ways to ensure that a book gets written to deadline, which is as follows:

- get organised
- get tough
- get help.

Getting organised

Try to establish a territory for writing your book. It could be a study (ideally), or a desk or surface in another room (better than nothing). If you are writing on a word processor, your space should ideally centre on the machine. If you are writing by hand or typewriter, you have more flexibility about where to settle. However, using the same place saves time, because you don't have to pack up after every session, and it helps you focus, psychologically, when you return to write some more.

Organising background materials, references, quotes and other essential pieces of information is very tedious at the time. However, it is really helpful when you are actually writing to be able to find and use a piece of information immediately, rather than having to stop to telephone the library or search a stack of journals. There are numerous ways of organising such material (*see* Box 13.1), and it doesn't matter which one or combination is used, provided that there is some method in the madness.

It is also very important to be organised about the business of writing a book. You will have a lot of correspondence with the publishers, the editor, and later the copy

---

Box 13.1: Ways of organising background materials

There is no single correct way to organise your materials, but many writers use a combination of the following:

- **card index box** – a cheap and easy method for keeping references/quotes together by subject. It is handy to have by the computer, but cannot be carried around. Carry spare cards instead, and add them later. This method is not suitable for whole articles, booklets or large pieces of information
- **exercise book** – cheap, convenient to carry around and not damaged by dropping! This method is good for references, quotes, information, etc., but is not suitable for whole articles
- **computer database** – handy for looking things up as you write without having to leave the computer; also stores a large amount of information in a small physical space, and is easy to search by text word. It cannot hold whole articles, etc. (unless these are scanned in). Instead, information has to be recorded elsewhere and transferred
- **filing cabinet** – more expensive, although second-hand cabinets are available. Can store articles, booklets etc., close to the desk, for consulting as you write. Easy to store by subject, but not suitable for 'small' pieces of information such as references.

---

editor, indexer and other individuals about your book. There is also the all-important contract, the instructions to authors and your proposal, which need to be consulted regularly as you produce the book. It is useful to start a file (a simple ringbinder is cheap and convenient) at the very beginning of the process, so that you can find and refer to these documents easily. If you are editing a book, or working with several co-authors, then dividing the file so that there is a section for your correspondence with each person involved will help you to keep track of each author's progress.

☞ **Keep some blank paper in the file for notes about telephone conversations with the editor. Many day-to-day decisions about the content, format and presentation of the book are made along the way through telephone contacts, and it is easy to forget what you agreed to do or include.**

A separate file, such as a box file or folder, is useful for keeping printouts of each chapter as you write it. It is much easier to consult a paper copy to check what you said in a previous chapter than to find the relevant passage in a computer file. A disk box solely for the disks containing book material is also advisable (imagine the nightmare of mislaying the disk with a whole section of the book on it).

☞ **If you are receiving disks containing material from co-authors or contributors,** make sure that you have a good virus-checking program installed on your computer (*see* Box 13.2).

Box 13.2:   A cautionary tale from my personal experience

With a deadline looming and eight chapters of a book on my computer, I used a disk from a contributor which turned out to have a virus on it. It corrupted the hard disk, which needed to be taken to a computer shop to be repartitioned before all of the programs I used could be reinstalled. Many expensive telephone calls to the software support company followed, and the computer is still not its old self today. 'But I have a virus checker on my computer,' I wailed to the man in the shop at the time. 'Hmmph,' he snorted. '*That* one's no good...'

Finally, of course, it helps to be organised about the act of writing. Everyone has their own way of writing, but I find the following principles helpful.

- Write a little every day or two, however small, because then you will feel that you are getting somewhere rather than feeling guilty all the time.
- Have breaks during longer writing spells, with incentives such as chocolate, alcohol or human company waiting for you at the end.
- Keep up the momentum when writing. Resist the urge to revise and rewrite every sentence as you go. Instead, reread the chapter or section as a whole later, and make revisions then.
- If you are writing on the word processor, save material very frequently (and/or use Autosave, set for every 5 minutes). Otherwise power cuts (or cats on the keyboard) can result in the loss of hours of work.
- Count the number of words in each chapter as it is written, for an estimate of a rough total as you go (although this will change with later revisions).
- Copy each session's work to disk when you stop, and use more than one disk for the book, in case one is damaged.
- Carry a notebook around with you for the moments when you suddenly realise what you missed out of Chapter 7 – then you don't have to go and alter it immediately, but can wait for your final revision.
- Use every opportunity, however short, to write or to plan your writing. Chapter plans can be written on trains or in waiting-rooms, and ideas for particular sections, approaches or phrases can be worked through while you are cooking, shopping or queuing.

☞ **If this sounds obsessive, it probably is – but writing a book is by no means a clinical and unemotional affair!**

GETTING TOUGH

There are two parts to this. First, you need to be tough with yourself, to make yourself write when you don't feel like it, or there is something 'unmissable' on television, or someone around you demands your attention. Then there is the really hard part – being tough on other people. Writing a book is like having a baby – it tends to alter your relationships with other people and, pleased as they are about your impending happy event, they tend to resent the intrusion into their previously settled lives. So you will find that people want you to go out or come downstairs, have a break or wash the car, when you are deep into chapter 9 and doing well. They may also see the book as something optional – something that you decided to do more or less on impulse, and which you could just stop if you wanted to.

☞ **The contract, timetable and list of milestones are your evidence in this situation. You need to convince the people around you that this book-writing is a serious business.**

GETTING HELP

Accept all the help you can get with your other responsibilities, because you are going to need every available moment to write the book. Getting help with housework or gardening, being driven instead of driving yourself, and sharing responsibility for ferrying children about, can all help here. None of this kind of help necessarily needs to be paid for (although if you can afford some extra help, that would be wonderful). Instead, the 'get tough' policy can be used to elicit help from previously disinterested family members or partners, to allow you more time to write. A useful phrase is 'The sooner it's finished, the sooner I can...'

KEEPING IN TOUCH WITH THE EDITOR

If writing a book is like having a baby, then your editor is the other parent. They have a responsibility to their company to ensure that the book they have commissioned actually arrives on time and as described in the proposal. After all, the company is going to invest much time and money in designing, producing, printing and marketing the book, and they have planned and budgeted for this. Failure to deliver would be like telling the grandparents who have already decorated the nursery and hand-built the cot that it was a phantom pregnancy after all.

It is essential to keep in touch with the editor during the writing of the book. In larger publishing companies, the commissioning editor may pass on responsibility for your book to a project editor. In smaller firms, the editor who commissioned the book may also maintain the contact through to publication. However, in either case, you will need to keep in touch in order to:

- reassure them that the book is progressing to plan (if it is)
- alert them if the book is falling behind schedule
- check any changes that you might want to make from the proposal
- discuss the effect of any new developments which might affect the topicality or relevance of your book
- talk about the marketing and promotion of your book.

DISPATCHING THE BOOK

Once the book has been written and final revisions have been incorporated, the final word count of each chapter can be made. If you have counted words as you go, and rechecked them after the revision of each chapter or section, then the total should not come as a surprise.

☞ **If the word count varies considerably from the length agreed to in the contract, talk to the editor before packing up the manuscript.**

Before packing up the manuscript, make a final check that all the publisher's instructions have been followed, and that the package is complete (*see* Box 13.3). Then the manuscript can be dispatched by registered post to the publisher.

The sense of relief and freedom once the project is off your hands is wonderful, and should be savoured for as long as possible. After a while, a sense of having 'nothing to do in the evenings' will creep in and, as with babies, the pain and pressure will be forgotten, and you will start to think about having another one.

WHAT HAPPENS NEXT?

Over a period of weeks or months, the publishers will copy edit your manuscript, producing a set of page proofs which look like the pages of the final book. While they are doing this, they may send you some queries to answer, or these may come to you with the proofs. Any diagrams and drawings in the manuscript will have been sent to an artist to reproduce, and they may also send queries related to these, with a copy of their version of the diagrams.

☞ **Treat all of these queries seriously and urgently – the publishers are working to a tight schedule to get your book out on time.**

The proofs themselves will be sent to you for correction – like article proofs, only

---

Box 13.3: Check-list for packaging a manuscript

Before dispatching the manuscript to the publisher, check that:

- the printouts are formatted as required (e.g. margins, headings, spacing, fonts, etc.)
- there is a hard copy of every chapter
- there is a copy of every chapter on disk
- all disks are labelled with your name, the book title, the contents and the name of the word-processing package you have used
- the disk and hard copies match exactly (i.e. they are the same version of the chapter)
- all tables, illustrations and photographs referred to in the text are included with the appropriate chapter
- all necessary permissions for use of copyright material have been obtained in writing and are included with the manuscript
- material for the 'prelims' (the preface, acknowledgements, details of your own and any contributors' degrees and appointments, and the contents list) is included.

---

much, much longer and more daunting! The editor will usually contact the author or editor before the proofs are sent, to say when they will arrive and to check that you are going to be available at that time to deal with them. The turnaround time on the proofs is usually about 2 weeks, so it is essential to set aside plenty of time to check them. The standard proof correction marks are shown in Appendix D.

☞ Be meticulous in checking every letter, diagram and label. They do sometimes get transposed, missed out or garbled during the typesetting process.

The proofs will usually also be checked by a professional proof-reader, who will look for 'literal' errors ('typos' which have been generated during the typesetting stage), but cannot check for errors of fact.

   While you are proof-reading, you may also be required to fill in cross-references to other pages in the book (full instructions will be sent with the proofs). If there are two sets of page proofs, one set (the 'master' or 'marked' set) should be returned to the publisher, while you keep the other set for your own reference.

☞ Corrections are very costly, and should be kept to essential corrections only. No new material can be added at the proof-reading stage.

The index for the book is usually prepared by a professional indexer, but you may be sent the index for comment, in case you think that an important topic has been missed out. This is usually the last contribution that you need to make to the production process.

Some time after this you will be sent a number of author's presentation copies of the finished book, as specified in the contract. These usually arrive shortly before the official publication date of the book. Then you can simply wait for the official date, and start looking for your book on the bookshop shelves and in the library catalogue.

☞ **The average time from delivery of the manuscript to the official publication date is about 1 year, although it can be as short as 6 months if the book is very topical and the publishers are keen to capitalise on this.**

SUMMARY

The key to success in writing a book is to start as soon as possible after the contract has been agreed and signed, and to measure your progress against some pre-set milestones. It is essential to be organised and disciplined in your approach to writing. When the publishers are in the process of producing your book, you will need to answer queries and check the page proofs swiftly and meticulously.

CHAPTER FOURTEEN

TOP TIPS FOR SUCCESS

If you have worked through this book from the beginning, you probably already have at least one completed article accepted for publication, and the hints and tips in this chapter will simply be reminders for the next piece you write.

If you have skipped straight to this chapter in your enthusiasm to start writing and being published, then you will find that it contains some terse instructions to maximise your chances of acceptance, but little in the way of helpful detail. That is contained in all of the previous chapters, which you might like to return to and read later on. For now, here are:

- ten *Rules of the Road* for writers
- five *Great Mistakes I Made* (but you needn't)
- ten *Frequently Asked Questions* (and their answers)
- some helpful *Words of Wisdom* from experienced journal editors.

RULES OF THE ROAD FOR WRITERS

1 Make sure someone is interested in your article/book before you write it.
2 Plan the article/book before you write it.
3 Keep sentences short and language simple.
4 Count words as you write each section.
5 Use minimum formatting, and follow the journal/publisher's guidelines.
6 Use plenty of subheadings to break up text in a journal article.
7 Use charts, graphs or figures rather than words to present numerical data.
8 Note down each reference in full as you use it.
9 Write at least a paragraph, and preferably a section, before revising and rewriting.
10 Send the finished work to only one journal/publisher at a time.

FIVE GREAT MISTAKES I MADE (BUT YOU NEEDN'T)

Mistake number 1: thinking no one but me and the editor actually read my piece

This was a comforting fallacy which allowed me to be lazy about checking facts, looking up references and searching for evidence. Unfortunately, it is not true. Many experts in the subject will read your article or book, and some of them are quite likely to write to you pointing out your errors and omissions.

Solution: be meticulous about checking facts, figures and references, but prepared to concede gracefully when – as inevitably happens sooner or later – you get it wrong.

Mistake number 2: being upset by criticism

Editors encourage individuality and even controversy, as this makes journals and books more interesting. Journal editors in particular are usually delighted if your opinion piece provokes a deluge of contributions to the letters page. However, letter writers can be savage in their criticism, and I often used to feel personally attacked and humiliated.

Solution: remember that you are entitled to express your own opinion, or to argue a particular viewpoint, and the reader is equally entitled to disagree. If critical letters continue to upset you, don't read the letters page.

Mistake number 3: assuming that the quality of my writing would compensate for poor presentation

I used to send articles to *Nursing Standard* that looked as if they had been left out in strong sunshine for a week before dispatch. John Naish, then editor of the Viewpoint section, sent me a plaintive note back with one cheque, saying 'Maybe you could treat your typewriter to a new ribbon...?' Fortunately he was patient enough to stick with me, but another editor might not have been so forbearing.

Solution: be professional about presentation from the start. Word-process your articles if at all possible, and use good-quality paper and strong envelopes.

Mistake number 4: sending articles to journals without assessing the journal first

The few rejections I have received in recent years have all stemmed from this one simple mistake. I am sure I have done my credibility no good with those journal editors by sending them inappropriate material, and it has wasted all the time and effort I put into writing the article in the first place.

Solution: either assess each new journal before you send a first article to them, or stick to writing for one or two journals that you know well.

Mistake number 5: being afraid to talk to editors

On several occasions I have sent articles to journals, only to have them praised but rejected because the editor already had something similar awaiting publication. I had not talked to the editor in advance, assuming that they would be too busy, important or intimidating to talk to me.

Solution: always telephone the editor or someone on the staff of the journal first. They are invariably friendly, approachable and helpful, and selling them the idea for an article makes it much more likely that it will eventually be published.

FREQUENTLY ASKED QUESTIONS

These are questions I am often asked either at Writing for Publication workshops or informally by colleagues. Some of them may be directly applicable to you, while others may spark a train of thought or a new question. If there are other questions to which you need answers, talk to the editor who is dealing with your article or book.

Question: I am a midwife, and I have always written about midwifery. Is there any chance of my getting an article accepted on a different subject, such as diabetes?

Answer: Yes, there is. Sharing expertise and information across different branches of the professions is recognised as being very important. If you look at the authors of articles in any professional journal, you will find a mixture of people contributing. You just need to explain to the editor why they should accept an article on diabetes from you – because you have done a course, studied it specifically, suffer from it, have an interest in it, or are writing about diabetes in pregnancy, etc.

Question: I have written an article for a journal which asks for a maximum of 2000 words per article. My piece is 3500 words and I really can't cover the subject in less. Should I send it in and see whether they will publish it as it is?

Answer: You could do that, but be prepared for them to return it to you for editing, or to edit it themselves, as they are not going to change the journal layout to accommodate your article. It would be better to telephone the editor to talk about it. You could suggest making it into two articles, or reducing the scope of the article so that you can cover the smaller subject in 2000 words.

Question: People say I have a good sense of humour, and I would like to write humorous pieces for a nursing journal, but I don't think I want to do this under my own name. Can I use a pseudonym?

Answer: It would be best to discuss this with the editor of the journal you are thinking of targeting. Some humorous articles, especially regular columns, are written under a heading rather than a name, or use what is clearly a '*nom de plume*', Sister Plume being one of the most famous of these.

Question: I have read that, to be taken seriously as a writer, one shouldn't try to sell a book idea to a publisher directly, but should use an agent. Is this correct?

Answer: In my experience it is not necessary to use an agent. With a limited amount of background work you can locate a suitable publisher, and the publishers themselves supply all of the guidance and help you could need to write a proposal.

Question: Can I negotiate the fee for my articles? I was recently paid £35 for 1000 words, which seems ridiculously small considering the amount of work I put in.

Answer: You cannot negotiate for uncommissioned articles, i.e. those sent following an expression of interest from an editor, or simply sent 'on spec'. You could try negotiating if the editor approaches you to write something, but the nursing journals don't have huge sums to pay out on fees, and the fee is unlikely to vary much. Some pay more than others, though, so you could try different journals, and then target the better payers in future.

Question: My articles always seem to be published under really silly titles, and never the title I gave them. Is there anything I can do about this?

Answer: Not really. Sub-editors think up titles, and they reflect the 'house style' of the journal, so if they favour punning or jokey headings, you are stuck with them.

Question: Who 'owns' the report that I wrote at work? Can I use it as the basis of an article without asking anyone?

Answer: Generally speaking, writing produced at work is the property of the company or employer. However, in the interests of professional development, most managers are keen for people to publish professional articles about their work, though it is sensible and courteous to ask if you can write up a particular project or piece of work, and obtain permission to use the report as a basis for it.

Question: My Family Planning Certificate isn't a recordable qualification. Does this mean that I can't put it down on the 'author's details' form, to go with my article on forms of contraception?

Answer: Do put it down on the form. It demonstrates that you have the expertise to write about the topic, which is the purpose of including the author's qualifications in the heading of the article.

Question: I have sent my book to the publisher, but I am really worried about having to proof-read it. What if I miss a mistake? Are they just relying on me to check the whole book?

Answer: Don't worry about proof-reading. You will be sent full instructions, and the correct use of the symbols quickly becomes ingrained as you work through the proofs. Set aside plenty of time to check them, and try to arrange to have some peace and quiet while you are doing this. Remember that the proofs will also be checked by a professional proof-reader, so typos and transposed figures, etc., should be spotted by them as well as by you.

Question: I don't have access to a computer, and I'm not very good at using one in any case. Can I write my articles on a typewriter?

Answer: Most of the journals will accept typed articles, although they prefer word-processed ones because they can then have a disk copy as well as a paper copy. If in doubt, talk to the editor of the journal you are targeting. If they insist on a word-processed article and a disk, ask if you can send the typewritten copy for their opinion. Then, if it is accepted for publication, you can pay someone to word-process it for you, and send in the disk.

WORDS OF WISDOM

Finally, here are some collected Words of Wisdom from editors. If you follow these, you stand a very good chance of finding an editor who is keen to publish your articles for years to come.

ON BEING APPROACHED BY POTENTIAL AUTHORS...

Clare Parker, Features Editor, *Practice Nurse*: 'I think it's a very good thing to do, we need to encourage it more. It helps if the person has a clear idea of what they're going to write, the key points they want to make. Then we can decide if it's appropriate for the journal.'

Judith Podmore, Editor, *Nursing Management*: 'Most editors would be happy to be rung up. It's better if they don't have an article ready – it's best to ring early on. Then the editor can say, "Focus on this aspect" or "This is what we need". People tend to ring too late on.'

Daniel Allen, Editor, *Mental Health Nursing*: 'I like authors who phone first. I know some people, including me, find this difficult. But if your carefully crafted article covers the same ground as another carefully crafted article the editor has just published, he or she is unlikely to want another on the same subject. If you send it in without checking, you may be wasting your time – and the editor's. On the phone, try to be brief, concise and friendly – even if the editor appears to be a grouchy old sod. Remember that this may be the start of a profitable relationship.'

ON THE MOST COMMON MISTAKES AUTHORS MAKE...

Clare Parker: 'Not following the house style. References are the big thing – without all the information requirements, they are no use to anybody. People using the wrong referencing method is a real pain.'

Judith Podmore: 'Not following the Guidelines for Contributors. If you follow those, you can't go far wrong – it cuts out at least half the mistakes. The worst offence some writers commit is not structuring their articles in a logical form: they just throw words down on paper. They should plan the structure before writing the article.'

Daniel Allen: 'Common mistakes include failing to read the journal, failing to think about the journal's readership, and ignoring the journal's Guidelines for Authors – most journals have these, and most authors ignore them. If you stick to the guidelines, you will keep on the right side of the editor and you will also understand the process your article goes through after you have sent it off. Another common mistake is writing in a strange pseudo-academic language which requires the use of five words where one will do. It may be an earth-inverting horticultural implement to you, but to everyone else it's a spade.'

ON THE MOST IRRITATING THINGS AUTHORS DO...

Daniel Allen:

- sending the same article to two or more journals at the same time: this is likely to get you added to the 'don't-touch-with-a-bargepole' list for many years to come
- assuming they have a right to be published
- ringing two days after sending off their article to ask what's happening
- inventing their own way to reference their article's 40 references
- ignoring the given word length
- giving an article a 15-word heading and then wondering why it has been changed
- missing a deadline.

ON TIPS FOR SUCCESS...

Clare Parker:

- be accommodating about changes: everything is peer reviewed, and changes are made with the best of intentions.

Daniel Allen:

- understand that an editor's job is to edit
- don't be wounded by rejection.

Judith Podmore:

- ring before you write
- stick to a clear writing style
- don't start an article with a quote!

ON WHAT MAKES AN EDITOR'S DAY...

Judith:

- a well-laid-out article, on a disk, which adheres to the guidelines and the word length, and talks about what it says it's about in the title
- an article I don't have to do anything with – but then I guess I'd be out of a job!

Clare:

- hearing from nurses in practice – especially if they've done some research
- someone coming up with a really innovative idea, on a really nitty-gritty area, and getting to the nub of the issue.

Daniel:

- a good article written to the specified length
- an article received before the given deadline
- 40 references listed in the correct house style
- an author who returns corrected proofs quickly
- an author who can be contacted
- an author who phones to say: 'Thanks for publishing my article. I thought the edited version looked great, and I'm really proud of it.'

APPENDIX A

ASSESSMENT OF SOME CURRENT JOURNALS

Journal	Readership	Sections	Other comments
Nursing Standard	General and specialist nurses, midwives and health visitors, nursing students	News, analysis, features, perspectives (including book and resource reviews), art and science (clinical), career development. Sister journals: *Elderly Care, Primary Health Care, Emergency Nurse, Nursing Management*	Runs 'continuing education' articles, with assessments, for distance learning; also has regular supplements on particular clinical topics (e.g. wound care, continence)
Nursing Times	General and specialist nurses, midwives and health visitors, nursing students	News, comment, Mediawatch, 'insight', practice. Sister journals: *NT Research, Community Nurse*	Runs 'study-hours' articles for distance learning; has regular clinical supplements
Journal of Clinical Nursing	Nursing, midwifery and health-visiting practitioners	Editorials, review articles, 'research in brief', book reviews	Articles are usually research reports or critical literature reviews

Journal	Readership	Sections	Other comments
Community Practitioner	Nurses and health visitors working in primary care	News, news features, professional, clinical, professional briefing, rights at work, resources, book reviews	Journal of the Community Practitioners' and Health Visitors' Association
Practice Nurse	Nurses working in general practice	News, analysis, professional development, clinical focus, book reviews	Also uses clinical quizzes and riddles
Journal of Clinical Excellence	Academics, professionals, clinicians and managers	Not yet established	Welcomes articles on clinical governance, National Health Service frameworks, clinical effectiveness, audit and professional development
Health Service Journal	Health service managers	News, news focus, opinion, features, book reviews	Features articles cover service delivery, projects and public health issues

REMINDERS ABOUT PUNCTUATION

THE COMMA ,

This should be used:

- to separate main clauses in a sentence (e.g. 'Type II diabetes, the commonest form, affects more older people than younger people')
- to avoid potential confusion in the sense of a sentence (e.g. 'During the night nurses monitor patients' recovery from surgery' would read more clearly if it was written, 'During the night, nurses monitor patients' recovery from surgery')
- to separate items in a list (e.g. 'Equipment needed includes a speculum, spatula, glass slide and fixative fluid').

It should not be used:

- to create very long sentences (e.g. 'Asthma is a very common condition, it is thought to affect between one in five and one in ten school children, they may sleep badly, have many days absence from school, be unable to join in games lessons and need frequent hospitalisations').

THE SEMICOLON ;

This should be used:

- to separate two or more clauses which are of equal importance, and which are linked by their content (e.g. 'Diabetes mellitus is caused by deficiency of insulin; diabetes insipidus is caused by deficiency of ADH').

It should not be used:

- to separate items in a list (e.g. 'Diabetic patients may undertake blood testing; urine testing; or both').

THE COLON :

This should be used:

- to introduce a list of items (e.g. 'Diabetes can have serious complications: neuropathy, blindness, nephropathy and foot disease')
- before a quotation (e.g. 'Lady Thatcher said: "The National Health Service is safe with us" ')
- to separate two clauses in a sentence, when the second clause is dependent on the first (e.g. 'The White Paper "The New NHS" focuses on primary care: this is where the most radical organisational change will take place').

THE APOSTROPHE '

This probably causes more anxiety and more red pencilling by editors than any other piece of punctuation. Keith Waterhouse used to write about the AAAA (the Association for the Abolition of the Aberrant Apostrophe), in recognition of people's tendency to insert apostrophes into their writing at random.

In fact, the apostrophe has only three simple uses:

- to indicate possession (e.g. the patient's leg, the doctor's opinion (or, in the plural, the patients' legs, the doctors' opinions))
- to indicate that one or more letters have been omitted (e.g. 'She'd left the ward' for 'She had left the ward')
- to enclose a quotation (e.g. E E Cummings wrote: 'We doctors know a hopeless case').

APPENDIX C

REFERENCING

The importance of complete and accurate references cannot be overemphasised. Editors will check every word, any missing information being notified to the author as a query, and it is much more difficult to fill in the details retrospectively than to do so at the time of writing. The reference list should be submitted on a separate page to the rest of the article.

FORMS OF REFERENCING

There are two main methods of referencing, namely the Vancouver method and the Harvard method.

The Vancouver method uses a number in superscript in the text, like this,[1] to indicate a reference. The reference list should contain each reference *numbered in the order in which it appears in the text.*

The Harvard method – which is becoming the most common method – denotes a reference in the text by the author's surname and the date of the publication cited, in parentheses, like this (Anderton, 1997).

The Guidelines for Contributors published by the journal or publisher will indicate which form of referencing they require.

Whichever method is used, every article reference in the list should contain:

- the author's surname and initials (e.g. Smith A B and Jones C D)
- the year of publication in parentheses (e.g. (1999))
- the title of the article (e.g. Treating dyspepsia following gastric surgery: research-based or a gut feeling?)
- the name of the journal in italics (e.g. *Journal of Post-Operative Excellence*)
- the volume, number and page range (e.g. Vol. 4 No. 13 pp. 15–20).

Example

Smith A B and Jones C D (1999) Treating dyspepsia following gastric surgery: research-based or a gut feeling? *Journal of Post-Operative Excellence* Vol. 4 No. 13 pp. 15–20.

Every book reference in the list should contain:

- the author's surname and initials (e.g. Brown E F and Green G H)
- the year of publication in parentheses (e.g. (1990))
- the title of the book in italics (e.g. *Morbid pathology for absolute beginners*)
- the place of publication (e.g. Edinburgh)
- the publisher of the book (e.g. Burke-Hare).

Example

Brown E F, Green G H, White I J (1990) *Morbid pathology for absolute beginners.* Edinburgh: Burke-Hare.

If the reference is to a chapter within a multi-authored book, then the reference list should show:

- the surname and initials of the author who wrote the chapter to which you are referring
- the full title of the chapter
- full details of the book in which the chapter appears.

Example

Shelley M (1990)* Pathology brought to life. In Brown E F and Green G H (Eds)** *Morbid pathology for absolute beginners.* Edinburgh: Burke-Hare.

* The date is the date of publication of the book as a whole, regardless of when the chapter might have been written.
** Eds: the editors' names are given as well as the chapter author's name.

VARIATIONS

There are some points on which even journals using the same referencing system differ in their conventions. For example, some will suggest that books with more than two authors should be cited as Brown *et al.*, 1996, both in the text and in the reference list, rather than giving all of the authors' names. Others will want the shortened '*et al.*' form in the text, but all authors' names to be cited in the reference list.

Journals also differ in their use of punctuation in the reference list, some using commas to divide parts of the reference, while others use colons, semi-colons or full stops. Some of them use bold type for volume numbers. To reproduce the exact requirements you should photocopy a reference list from an existing article in your targeted journal and use it as a guide. However, it is not something to worry about too much, as the journal's sub-editor will ensure that the house style is followed. What is vitally important is that you provide all of the necessary information for the reference.

USEFUL POINTERS

- Get into the habit of noting down the reference in the form in which it will finally appear at the time when you note the quote or statistic you are intending to use. This is good practice for writing reference lists, and it also ensures that you will have all of the information you need.
- In some journals the full reference of the article is printed either beneath the title of the article or at the foot of the first page. Photocopy the page to save time and errors made by hand copying.
- References should be made to primary sources whenever possible, i.e. if an author quotes a figure for the incidence of single parenthood, citing the decennial census as the source, and you want to use that statistic, you should cite the census, not the author of the piece in which you read this. The key question to ask is: 'Is it *the author's* information?' It is the author's information if:

  - it is their opinion
  - it is taken from their research, audit or project
  - they are commenting, or making an assertion.

In this case, you should cite the author of the article when referring to this information. It is *not* the author's information if:

  - it is a statistic taken from another source
  - it is a fact taken from another person's work, research or article
  - it is a generally accepted piece of knowledge.

In this case, you should cite the original source, work or article.

SUGGESTED TEMPLATES FOR ARTICLES

Type of article	Suggested headings (indicative content)
Clinical, descriptive	Introduction (aim of the article)
	Background to issue/condition (definition, size, severity, impact, morbidity, etc.)
Aim: to educate or assist revision	The condition/issue (description of disease process and effect, or description of the issue)
Example topics:	Treatments/tackling the issue (medical, surgical, pharmaceutical, behavioural, practice, service change, etc.)
• asthma in adolescents	Professional issues involved
• postnatal depression	An example in practice [in box/side panel]
• urinalysis	Summary
• nasogastric feeding	
• stroke rehabilitation	

Project report

    Aim: to share good/innovative practice

    Example topics:
- setting up a carers' group
- introducing clinical supervision
- formulating leg ulcer treatment guidelines
- using significant event audit in palliative care

Introduction (aim of the article)

Background to the project (idea, impetus, funding)

Context for the project (how things were before the project, background to the issue)

Getting started (who led, how planning was carried out, obstacles encountered)

Implementing the project (experience of setting up)

The project in practice (findings, impact, effect on participants and others, lessons learned)

Future plans (how project will continue or expand)

Professional, discussion

    Aim: to assist in professional development

    Example topics:
- returning to practice
- confidentiality and electronic patient data
- record-keeping in the community
- violence against nurses in Accident and Emergency departments

Introduction (aim of the article)

Background to the issue (who/how many nurses it affects, how it affects patients, why it is important)

Exploring the issue (facts and figures, different opinions/perspectives)

Tackling the issue (what has been tried in the past, new ideas about dealing with it)

Topical example from practice [box or side panel]

Summary

Audit report

    Aim: to share findings and improve practice

    Example topics:
- audit of palliative care against national guidelines
- audit of leg ulcer treatment against proposed new guidelines
- audit of nurses' qualifications for giving advice on contraception

Introduction (aim of article)

Background to the topic (importance of topic, effect on patients)

The standard (whose standard, how it was found, what it says)

Carrying out the audit (how it was done, difficulties, limitations)

Findings (how practice compared with the standards used)

Implications for practice (what changes, education, etc. were necessary)

Re-audit (findings from second audit)

Conclusion

Research report

Aim: to share findings

Example topics:
- survey of doctors' views on nurse practitioners
- content analysis of nurses' notes in palliative care
- case–control study of aromatherapy in treatment of mild depression

Introduction (purpose of article)
Background (to the issue)
Literature review (summary of previous research on the topic, critical discussion of methodologies, relevance, etc.)
Aim (of research described)
Method (of research described)
Findings (tables, figures, charts, description)
Discussion (of validity and relevance of finding, implications for practice)
Limitations (of study, due to methodology or other factors)
Conclusion

PROOF CORRECTION SYMBOLS

Group A   General

Number	Instruction	Textual mark	Marginal mark	Notes
A1	Correction is concluded	None	/	P Make after each correction
A2	Leave unchanged	– – – – – – under characters to remain	(✓)	M P
A3	Remove extraneous marks	Encircle marks to be removed	✕	P e.g. film or paper edges visible between lines on bromide or diazo proofs
A3.1	Push down risen spacing material	Encircle blemish	⊥	P
A4	Refer to appropriate authority anything of doubtful accuracy	Encircle word(s) affected	(?)	P

Group B   Deletion, insertion and substitution

Number	Instruction	Textual mark	Marginal mark	Notes
B1	Insert in text the matter indicated in the margin	⋏	New matter followed by ⋏	M P Identical to B2
B2	Insert additional matter identified by a letter in a diamond	⋏	⋏ Followed by for example ⟨A⟩	M P The relevant section of the copy should be supplied with the corresponding letter marked on it in a diamond e.g. ⟨A⟩
B3	Delete	/ through character(s) or ⊢——⊣ through words to be deleted	∂	M P
B4	Delete and close up	⌢/⌣ through character or ⊂——⊃ through character e.g. charac̑ter charac̑ter	∂̑	M P

Number	Instruction	Textual mark	Marginal mark	Notes
B5	Substitute character or substitute part of one or more word(s)	/ through character or ⊢————⊣ through word(s)	New character or new word(s)	M P
B6	Wrong fount. Replace by character(s) of correct fount	Encircle character(s) to be changed	⊗	P
B6.1	Change damaged character(s)	Encircle character(s) to be changed	✕	P This mark is identical to A3
B7	Set in or change to italic	———— under character(s) to be set or changed	⊔⊔	M P Where space does not permit textual marks encircle the affected area instead
B8	Set in or change to capital letters	≡≡≡ under character(s) to be set or changed	≡	
B9	Set in or change to small capital letters	══ under character(s) to be set or changed	══	
B9.1	Set in or change to capital letters for initial letters and small capital letters for the rest of the words	≡≡ under initial letters and ══ under rest of word(s)	≡	
B10	Set in or change to bold type	∿∿∿∿ under character(s) to be set or changed	∿	
B11	Set in or change to bold italic type	∿∿∿∿ under character(s) to be set or changed	⊔⊔∿	
B12	Change capital letters to lower case letters	Encircle character(s) to be changed	≢	P For use when B5 is inappropriate
B12.1	Change small capital letters to lower case letters	Encircle character(s) to be changed	≢	P For use when B5 is inappropriate

Number	Instruction	Textual mark		Marginal mark	Notes
B13	Change italic to upright type	Encircle character(s) to be changed		⊔	P
B14	Invert type	Encircle character to be inverted		↻	P
B15	Substitute or insert character in 'superior' position	/	through character	˥	P
		or ∧	where required	under character e.g. ⌄2	
B16	Substitute or insert character in 'inferior' position	/	through character	L	P
		or ∧	where required	over character e.g. ⌐2	
B17	Substitute ligature e.g. ffi for separate letters	├─────┤ through characters affected		⌢ e.g. ffi	P
B17.1	Substitute separate letters for ligature	├─────┤		Write out separate letters	P
B18	Substitute or insert full stop or decimal point	/	through character	⊙	M P
		or ∧	where required		
B18.1	Substitute or insert colon	/	through character	⊙	M P
		or ∧	where required		
B18.2	Substitute or insert semi-colon	/	through character	;	M P
		or ∧	where required		
B18.3	Substitute or insert comma	/	through character	,	M P
		or ∧	where required		

Number	Instruction	Textual mark		Marginal mark	Notes
B18.4	Substitute or insert apostrophe	/	through character	ᛉ	M P
		or			
		⋏	where required		
B18.5	Substitute or insert single quotation marks	/	through character	ᛉ and/or ᛉ	M P
		or			
		⋏	where required		
B18.6	Substitute or insert double quotation marks	/	through character	ᛉ and/or ᛉ	M P
		or			
		⋏	where required		
B19	Substitute or insert ellipsis	/	through character	• • •	M P
		or			
		⋏	where required		
B20	Substitute or insert leader dots	/	through character	(•••)	M P Give the measure of the leader when necessary
		or			
		⋏	where required		
B21	Substitute or insert hyphen	/	through character	⊢—⊣	M P
		or			
		⋏	where required		
B22	Substitute or insert rule	/	through character	⊢—⊣	M P Give the size of the rule in the marginal mark e.g. ⊢1 em⊣ ⊢4 mm⊣
		or			
		⋏	where required		
B23	Substitute or insert oblique	/	through character	(/)	M P
		or			
		⋏	where required		

Group C Positioning and spacing

Number	Instruction	Textual mark	Marginal mark	Notes
C1	Start new paragraph	⌐_	⌐_	M P
C2	Run on (no new paragraph)	⌒	⌒	M P
C3	Transpose characters or words	⎣⎤ between characters or words, numbered when necessary	⎣⎤	M P
C4	Transpose a number of characters or words	**3 2 1** | | |	**1 2 3**	M P To be used when the sequence cannot be clearly indicated by the use of C3. The vertical strokes are made through the characters or words to be transposed and numbered in the correct sequence
C5	Transpose lines	S	S	M P
C6	Transpose a number of lines		——— 3 ——— 2 ——— 1	P To be used when the sequence cannot be clearly indicated by C5. Rules extend from the margin into the text with each line to be transplanted numbered in the correct sequence
C7	Centre	⌐enclosing matter to be centred⌐	[ ]	M P
C8	Indent	⌐	⌐	P Give the amount of the indent in the marginal mark
C9	Cancel indent	←⌐	⌐	P
C10	Set line justified to specified measure	←⌐ and/or ⌐→	←→	P Give the exact dimensions when necessary

Number	Instruction	Textual mark	Marginal mark	Notes
C11	Set column justified to specified measure	⊢——→	⊢→	M P Give the exact dimensions when necessary
C12	Move matter specified distance to the right	enclosing matter to be moved to the right →		P Give the exact dimensions when necessary
C13	Move matter specified distance to the left	← enclosing matter to be moved to the left		P Give the exact dimensions when necessary
C14	Take over character(s), word(s) or line to next line, column or page			P The textual mark surrounds the matter to be taken over and extends into the margin
C15	Take back character(s), word(s), or line to previous line, column or page			P The textual mark surrounds the matter to be taken back and extends into the margin
C16	Raise matter	over matter to be raised under matter to be raised		P Give the exact dimensions when necessary. (Use C28 for insertion of space between lines or paragraph in text)
C17	Lower matter	over matter to be lowered under matter to be lowered		P Give the exact dimensions when necessary. (Use C29 for reduction of space between lines or paragraphs in text)
C18	Move matter to position indicated	Enclose matter to be moved and indicate new position		P Give the exact dimensions when necessary
C19	Correct vertical alignment	‖	‖	P
C20	Correct horizontal alignment	Single line above and below misaligned matter e.g. mi$_s$align$_e$d		P The marginal mark is placed level with the head and foot of the relevant line

Number	Instruction	Textual mark	Marginal mark	Notes
C21	Close up. Delete space between characters or words	linking ⌒ characters	⌒	M P
C22	Insert space between characters	| between characters affected	Y	M P Give the size of the space to be inserted when necessary
C23	Insert space between words	Y between words affected	Y	M P Give the size of the space to be inserted when necessary
C24	Reduce space between characters	| between characters affected	⋂	MP Give the amount by which the space is to be reduced when necessary
C25	Reduce space between words	⋂ between words affected	⋂	M P Give amount by which the space is to be reduced when necessary
C26	Make space appear equal between characters or words	| between characters or words affected	⟊	M P
C27	Close up to normal interline spacing	(each side of column linking lines)		MP The textual marks extend into the margin
C28	Insert space between lines or paragraphs	⊢⟨ or ⟨⊣		M P The marginal mark extends between the lines of text. Give the size of the space to be inserted when necessary
C29	Reduce space between lines or paragraphs	⟶⟩ or ⟵⊏		M P The marginal mark extends between the lines of text. Give the amount by which the space is to be reduced when necessary

APPENDIX F

A QUICK GUIDE TO THE INTERNET AND THE WORLD WIDE WEB

There are many reasons why writers might want to use the Internet or the World Wide Web (WWW) – finding references, searching databases, reading 'on-line' journals, accessing policy documents, exchanging views and information with other professionals, and simply using electronic mail (email) are just some of them. This very brief and simple guide is an introduction for the uninitiated.

- The **Internet** is a world-wide network of computers linked by telephone lines. To use the Internet you need a computer, a telephone line, a modem and an Internet service provider.
- A **modem** is a device, either internal to your computer or consisting of an external box, which converts digital signals from your computer into a form that can be sent down a telephone line.
- An **Internet service provider** is a company that sells you a connection to the Internet, giving you access to the World Wide Web, email and other services for the price of a local telephone call.
- The **World Wide Web** provides a way of looking around the information that is available on the Internet, using a Web 'browser', which is a software program that displays Web pages on the computer screen, and links to other pages. A 'search engine' is a program which helps with searches by tracking information using the key words or subject categories you provide.
- An **online service provider** makes access to the Internet easier by organising the information available. In effect, your Internet service provider gives you the key to

the door of a huge library, while the online service provider, inside the door, is your guide round the rooms, shelves and catalogues.

- The **NHSnet** is an 'intranet', a kind of mini-Internet solely for NHS users. It contains several 'zones' of information, including a clinical zone, an IM&T zone, an information zone for news on the NHS and health, and an executive zone. It also gives access to a number of databases for searches, as well as providing an email service.

There are many opportunities to learn how to use the Internet and the World Wide Web, including:

- training at work, as part of the national information strategy
- free demonstrations and training offered by local authorities, often in public libraries and careers offices
- training by library staff at professional organisations' resource centres
- training by university library or information staff, for students on postgraduate courses.

It is becoming more and more important for writers to be able to find and use information that is available on the Internet, and to communicate via email. It is worth the initial effort of finding and taking up training opportunities to be able to do these things.

SAMPLE RECORD SHEET FOR WRITING INCOME

Date sent	Title	Number of words	Journal	Payment	Date received	Declared for tax
28/01/98	Testing children's hearing	1500	*Nursing Standard*	£60	11/7/98	Yes

INDEX

abstracts 130
academic texts 149
acceptance
  of articles 83–5
  of ideas 43
acceptance letters 83–4
  payment rates 90
acknowledgements
  for previously published material 69
  of receipt of article by journal 81
agents 168
aims of book 148–9
American English v. British English 6, 65
anniversaries, linking topics to 38–9
  humorous writing 119
anonymous columns 111, 167
apostrophe 176
appendices 150
approaches
  of articles 62–4
    v. dissertations 124
    series 108
  of books 148–9
  to editors 35, 45–6, 169
    from dissertation to article 129–30
    humorous writing 120–1
    outcome 42–5
    phone call 40–2
    preparation 36–40
    reasons for 35–6, 167
  of journals 31, 62

  to publishers 142–3
  to writing a book 156–7
articles
  references to 177–8
  writing see writing articles
assessment of journals 25–7
  approach of articles 62–3
  contents 30–2
  contributors 29–30
  from dissertation to article 27–8
  importance 166
  readership 27–9
audit reports 182
author's details forms 84–5, 168

background materials, organising 158, 159
background of book 144
blurbs 151
bold type 61
books
  references to 178
  reviews 100–1, 111
  writing see writing books
boxes, list of 61
brand names of drugs 65–6
British English v. American English 6, 65
British Journal of Community Nursing 28
browsers, World Wide Web 193

card index boxes 159
career advancement 98

Centre for Evidence-Based Medicine 101
chapters
    in multi-authored books, contributing
        136–9
    contents list, book proposal 150
circulation of weeklies 3–4
clinical articles
    regular 103–5
    template 181
Clinical Guidelines Index 101
co-authors 73
collaborating
    articles 72–3
    books 136–9, 150
colon 176
columns, regular 109–10
    anonymous 111
    content 110
    and proof-reading 85
comma 175
comments after publication 91–2
    see also readers' letters
commission 138
commissioning editors 136, 137, 140
    approaching 143
    keeping in touch with 161–2
    proposals 152–3
    word length, advice on 150
commissioning letters
    articles 44
        payment rates 90
    books, multi-authored 138
commissioning of articles 43
Community Nurse 94
Community Practitioner 94, 174
    contents 174
    example article 131
    readership 27, 174
Community Practitioners' and Health
    Visitors' Association 94
competing texts 146–8
complementary texts 146–8
complimentary copies
    of book 164
    of journal 86, 89–90
computers

databases 159
floppy disks
    articles 60, 77–9, 169
    books 159–60, 163
formatting articles 61
v. paper 58–9
pie charts and graphs 65
saving material 160
spelling and grammar correction 6, 65
word-processing 60, 79, 87, 168–9
conferences, national nursing 101–2
consequences of publication 9
contacts 95–6
contents
    of articles
        agreeing with editor 43, 45
        regular columns 110
    of books 150
    of journals 30–2, 173–4
        assessing target readership 27–9
        recent coverage of topic 31–2
contracts, book 153
contributors
    to articles 73
    to books 136–9, 150
    to journals 29–30
copies of articles 86, 89–90
copy editing 162
copyright 8
    forms 84
corrections
    to proofs
        articles 85–6
        books 163, 168
        proof-reading symbols 186–92
    for reprinting 95
covering letters 80, 87
    humorous articles 120
credibility
    academic/professional 97
        weekly journals 3
    with editor and journal staff 123
        knowing the journals 23
criticism 91–3, 121–2, 166
cross-references 163
CV 98

deadlines
  for articles
    agreeing 44
    approaching the editor 40
    missed 45, 170
  for books 153, 157
  for proof-reading corrections
    articles 85
    books 163
  for sections, self-imposed 57–8
Department of Health Home Page 101
descriptive articles 181
Diabetic Medicine 31
diagrams, list of 61
diaries 110
directories 149
discussion articles 182
disk copies
  of articles 60, 77–9, 169
  of books 159–60, 163
dispatching
  articles 79–81
    preparation 77–9
  books 162, 163
dissertations 123, 126–9, 132–3
  material to save 125–6
  planning the article 130–1, 132
  reasons for publication 124–5
  talking to the editor 129–30
  writing the article 131
drawings, use of 63
drugs
  doses 66
    proof-reading 85
  names 65–6

editorial board 152
editors, book 138, 139
editors, commissioning 136, 137, 140
  approaching 143
  keeping in touch with 161–2
  proposals 152–3
  word length, advice on 150
editors, journal
  approaching 35, 45–6, 169
    from dissertation to article 129–30

humorous writing 120–1
  outcome 42–5
  phone call 40–2
  preparation 36–40
  reasons for 35–6, 167
credibility with 23
deadline problems 45
defining the topic 12, 15
details about 29, 39
information needed from 39–40
revision process 83
'selling' your ideas to 12, 18, 40, 41
series 108
weeklies 3
editors, project 161–2
educational articles
  collaborating 72
  planning 51–2
Elderly Care 94, 173
email 80, 193, 194
Emergency Nurse 94, 173
English as second language 68
entertaining articles 21–2
  see also humorous writing; quizzes
'et al.', use of 178
exercise books 159
  for ideas 117, 160
  for organisation 159
expert, writing as a 103, 104

fame 97
fastening pages 79
faxing of articles 80
fees
  for articles 90, 97
    negotiations 168
    reprints 95
    sample record sheet 195
  for books 138
figures (drawings)
  list of 61
  presentation 61
  use of 63, 65
figures (numbers) 66
filing cabinets 159
filing systems

articles 99, 100, 102
books 159
finding journals 24–5
finding publishers 141–2
floppy disks
articles 60, 77–9, 169
books 159–60, 163
fonts 61
formality of style, degree of 64
formatting
of articles 61
of books 155–6, 163
forms of writing 20, 21

galley proofs 85
gender-neutral language 68
generalist, writing as a 103, 104–5
generic drug names 65
ghost writers 73
grammar 5–6, 175–6
graphs, use of 63, 64, 65
Guidelines for Contributors/Authors
articles 3
approaching the editor 40
approach of articles 62, 63
copying 31
following advice 7, 169–70
language 68
lengths of articles 40, 44
numbers 66
obtaining 31, 40
presentation of articles 60, 61
submission 77, 79
books 155–6

handbooks 149
hard copies
articles 77, 79
books 163
Harvard referencing method 177
headings, section 49, 63
formatting 61
'invisible' 53
research reports 63
Healthgate 101
Health Service Journal 174

anonymous columns 111
approach of articles 62
contents 174
humorous writing 114
readership 174
Health Services Research Super Highway
101
help 161
house style 61, 169–70
see also Guidelines for Contributors/
Authors
humorous writing 113, 121–2
approach 63
approaching the editor 120–1
defining the topic 21–2
fitting material to journals 7
getting started 115–19
knowing the journal 119–20
opportunities 113–15
and proof-reading 85
proposals 38
pseudonyms 111, 167
style 64
weekly journals 3
writing the piece 121

income from writing 90, 97
reprints 95
sample record sheet 195
see also fees
indentations 61
indexes 163–4
informality of style, degree of 64–5
information resources 99, 100, 101
Internet 99, 193–4
Internet service providers 193–4
italic type 61

job prospects 97, 98
Journal of Clinical Excellence 174
Journal of Clinical Nursing 129, 173
contents 31, 173
mission statement 28
readership 173
journals *see* knowing the journals
justifying text 61

key words 130
knowing the journals 32–3
    assessing 25–7
        approach of articles 62–3
        contents 30–2
        contributors 29–30
        from dissertation to article 127–8
        importance 166
        readership 27–9
knowing the publishers 141–2

'ladder', writing 12
language
    English as second 68
    formality and informality 64–5, 170
    gender-neutral 68
    see also style of writing
layout and presentation 166
    of articles 60–2, 171
    of books 155–6, 163
lead authors 73
lead times 39
learning, humour as 113, 114
lengths
    of articles
        checking with editor 40, 44
        counting words 59
        v. dissertation/project report lengths 124
        journal's requirements 7, 167, 170
        opinion pieces 7
    of books 150, 160, 162
    of sections 50
    of sentences 64
letters
    acceptance 83–4
        payment rates 90
    commissioning
        articles 44, 90
        books 138
    covering 80, 87
        humorous articles 120
    readers' 91–3, 166
        about humorous articles 122
letters pages 91
libraries 99, 101

managers
    copies of article 90
    permission to write article 50, 69, 75
margins 61
market for book 144–5
media reviews 111
Memorandum of Agreement 153
milestones, writing a book 157
mission statements of journals 27, 28
modems 193
multidisciplinary journals 128–9
multiple authors
    articles 72–3
    books 136–9, 150
    referencing 178
myths about writing 1–7

names of patients/clients 68
narrative humorous writing 118
national nursing conferences 101–2
NHSnet 194
notebooks
    for ideas 117, 160
    for organisation 159
NT Research 94, 173
    mission statement 28
numbering of pages 61, 79
numbers 66
numerical data 65, 66
Nurse WWW Information Service 101
Nursing Management 94, 173
Nursing Standard 173
    anonymous columns 111
    contents 2, 28, 173
    humorous writing 111, 113–14, 119
    readership 173
    'sister' publications 3, 94, 173
Nursing Times 173
    anonymous columns 111
    contents 173
    contributors 29, 30
    humorous writing 111, 113–14, 119
    mission statement 28
    readership 173
    'sister' publications 3, 94, 173

offers of work 106–8
    contributing to multi-author books 136–7
    regular columns 109
offprints of article 86, 89, 90
online service providers 193–4
opinion pieces
    length 7
    planning 53–4
    and proof-reading 85
    proposals 38, 39
    regular 105–6
    style 64
    weekly journals 3
organisation
    regular article writing 99, 100, 102
    writing a book 158–60
outline of book 144

pacing, writing a book 157
page proofs
    articles 85
    books 162–3
paper
    v. computer 58–9
    quality 79
paper clips 79
paragraphs 66
    formatting 61
Patient Information web site 101
patients
    names 68
    permission to write article 50, 68–9
payment
    for articles 90, 97
        negotiations 168
        reprints 95
        sample record sheet 195
    for books 138
peer reviews *see* reviews, prior to publication
percentages 66
permission
    to reproduce published material 69, 79,
        84, 163
    to write article 50, 68–9, 75, 168
Personal Professional Profiles 89, 98
perspective pieces, humorous 118

photographs
    submission 77, 79
    use of 63
picture libraries 79
pie charts, use of 65
plagiarism 69
planning
    articles 47–8, 54–5
        defining the topic 11
        from dissertations 130–1, 132
        steps 48–54
    books 140–1, 160
posting
    articles 79–81
    books 162
post-registration education and practice
    (PREP) programme 98
Practice Manager 27
Practice Nurse 174
    anonymous columns 111
    contents 174
    humorous writing 114
    readership 27, 174
prelims 163
presentation 166
    of articles 60–2, 171
    of books 155–6, 163
presentation copies of books 164
Primary Health Care 94, 173
    example article 69
Primary Health Care Research and Development
    129
    approach of articles 62
    target readership 27
professional advancement 98
professional articles
    regular 103–5
    template 182
project descriptions
    collaborating 72
    colleagues' opinions 75
    from dissertation to article 126
    lengths 124
    planning 50–1
    template 182
project editors 161–2

proof-reading
  articles 85–6
  books 163, 168
  symbols 186–92
proposals
  articles 37–9
  books 140, 142–53
    multi-authored 137
pseudonyms 111, 167
publishers
  approaching 142–3
  knowing 141–2
punctuation 6, 61, 66, 175–6
  in reference lists 178–9
puzzles 111

queries
  after publication 91–2
  prior to publication 85
quizzes 111, 114
  defining the topic 20

readership
  articles 3–4, 173–4
    assessing target readership 27–9
    defining 14, 15, 16, 17
    from dissertation to article 127
    existence of 166
    finding the journals 24
    targeting 11
  books 144–5
readers' letters 91–3, 166
  about humorous articles 122
recorded delivery 81
refereeing process see reviews, prior to
    publication
reference books 99, 101
references 66–8, 170, 177–9
  forms 177–9
  list 61, 68, 177
  noting in full 60, 67–8, 179
regular writing 97–8, 111–12
  clinical/professional articles 103–5
  columns 109–10
    anonymous 111
    content 110

  and proof-reading 85
  ground rules 98
  offers of work 106–8
  opinion articles 105–6, 107
  options 102, 111
  same v. different journals 106, 107
  series, writing for a 108–9
  starting out 99–102
rejections
  articles 170
    humorous writing 121
    of initial ideas 42–3
    reasons for 5, 8
    and sending articles 'on the rounds' 4
    and targeting journals 23, 24
    time between submissions and 8
  book proposals 152–3
reports as basis for articles 168
reprints 84, 94–5
research 97
  see also dissertations
research reports
  format 129, 130
  subheadings 63
  template 183
reviewers as collaborators 73
reviews
  of books 100–1
  of media 111
  prior to publication 81–2, 170
    book proposals 152
    poorly planned/unplanned articles 48
    and sending articles 'on the rounds' 4, 5
  of television 111
revisions
  articles 58, 82–3, 87
    poorly planned/unplanned 48
    requests as conditional acceptance 5
    and sending articles 'on the rounds' 4, 5
  books 156–7
'rounds', sending articles on the 4, 5
royalties 138

salami publishing 127
satire 118–19
'scans' of journals 111

scope of book 148–9
search engines, World Wide Web 193
secondary markets for books 145
sections of article
    headings 49, 63
        formatting 61
        'invisible' 53
        research reports 63
    lengths 50
    planning 49–50
        from dissertation 130–1
semicolon 175–6
sentence length 64
series, writing for a 108–9
spacing of text 61
specialist, writing as a 103, 104
spelling 6, 65
spoof items 118
staff, journal 29
    credibility with 23
    see also editors, journal
staples, avoidance of 79
starting to write
    articles 57–8
        humorous writing 115–19
    books 135–6, 139–40, 155–6
style
    of articles 57, 64–5
        v. dissertations 124
        series 108
    of books 148–9
    of journals 31
sub-editors 83
subheadings 49, 63
    formatting 61
    'invisible' 53
    research reports 63
submitting articles
    to one journal at a time 8, 80, 170
    of unpublished material only 8
subscriptions to journals 99–100

tables, use of 63, 64
tabulation 61
taxation 90, 100
technical aspects of writing 65–9

television reviews 111
templates for articles 181–3
time factors
    articles
        approaching the editor 36
        proof-reading 85
        publication process 8
        readers' letters, replies to 91
        rejection 8, 24
        series 109
        topicality 38–9
        writing process 6–7
    books
        publication process 145–6, 164
        topicality 145, 146
        writing 155, 157, 158
title page 61, 62
titles
    of articles 62, 168, 170
    of sections 49, 63
        formatting 61
        'invisible' 53
        research reports 63
topicality
    of articles 38–9
        opinion pieces 105
    of books 146
topics
    articles
        from dissertations 126–7
        humorous pieces 117
        identifying 11–22
        new angles on 32
        recent coverage of 31–2
    books 140–1
toughness 161
typing of manuscript 60, 168–9

UKCC booklets 99, 101
underlining 61

Vancouver referencing method 177
virus checkers 160
voluntary organisations 102

web browsers 193

web sites 100, 101
  reviews 111
weekly journals 3–4
Word 6
word count *see* lengths
word-processing of manuscript 60, 79, 87,
    168–9
workbooks 149
World Health Organisation 101
World Wide Web (WWW) 99, 193–4
  browsers 193
  sites 100, 101
    reviews 111
Writers' and Artists' Yearbook 141
writing ability 5–6
writing articles 57, 73–5
  approach 62–4
  collaborating 72–3
  from dissertations 131
  examples 69–72
  humour 121

practicalities
    getting started 57–8
    paper v. computer 58–60
    presentation 60–2
  style 64–5
  technicalities 65–9
writing books 135, 153–4, 155, 162–4
  approaches to 156–7
  approaching the publishers 143
  dispatching the book 162, 163
  editors, keeping in touch with 161–2
  getting started 135–6, 139–40, 155–6
  help 161
  knowing the publishers 141–2
  managing your life 158
  organisation 158–60
  planning the topic 140–1
  proposals 143–52
    responses to 152–3
  timing and pacing 157
  toughness 161